Starting Monday

*Seven Keys to a Permanent, Positive
Relationship with Food*

Karen R. Koenig, LCSW, M.Ed

gürze books

Starting Monday
Seven Keys to a Permanent, Positive Relationship with Food

© 2013 by Karen R. Koenig, LCSW, M.Ed

Gürze Books
P.O. Box 2238
Carlsbad, CA 92018
760-434-7533
www.gurzebooks.com

Cover design by Johnson Design
www.toprotype.com
Author photo by Sue Messina
www.suemessinaphotography.com

Library of Congress Cataloging-in-Publication Data

Koenig, Karen R., 1947-
Starting Monday : seven keys to a permanent, positive relationship
with food / Karen R. Koenig, LCSW, Med.
    pages cm
ISBN 978-0-936077-78-9 (trade pbk. : alk. paper) --
ISBN 978-0-936077-79-6 (ebook)
1. Nutrition. 2. Diet. 3. Food habits. I. Title.
RA784.K548 2013
613.2--dc23
                            2013023383

NOTE:
The author and publisher of this book intend for this publication to
provide accurate information. It is sold with the understanding that it
is meant to complement, not substitute for, professional medical and/or
psychological services.

1 3 4 5 9 0 8 6 4 2

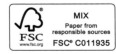

To my husband, Keith: I will never run out of thanks.

CONTENTS

Challenges to "Normal" Eating

The Seven Keys

Moving Forward

ACKNOWLEDGEMENTS

Many thanks to Janice M. Pieroni, my agent, for believing in the ideas behind this book throughout its several incarnations. And likewise to my publishers at Gürze Books, Leigh and Lindsey Cohn, for making this project so much fun to do, and to Leigh in particular for helping me keep it simple.

"People often have strong defense mechanisms that keep them rooted in their old habits. Defense mechanisms can operate below the level of conscious thought, allowing you to dismiss information before it threatens your world view."

> – Linda Bacon, Ph.D
> *Health at Every Size: The Surprising Truth about Your Weight*

"Only when you have gone sufficiently deep into your conflict do you understand its necessity."

> – Thomas Moore, Ph.D
> *Dark Nights of the Soul: A Guide to Finding Your Way Through Life's Ordeals*

INTRODUCTION

If you're reading this book, I'm guessing you've been wrestling with food for ages, even for what seems like—or has been—a lifetime. If so, hats off to you for persisting in trying to improve your eating and become healthier when the process, at times, may have felt frustrating, overwhelming, difficult, and as if it's hardly worth the effort. I'm here to tell you it *is* worth the effort, but only when you're heading down the right path.

Most disregulated eaters have had more than enough dead-end excursions into dieting, weight obsession, and the various and sundry ways of beating their appetites into submission and their bodies into shape. In fact, you could probably receive an honorary degree in nutrition from all the do's and don'ts you've learned about eating and could enjoy a splurge on Rodeo Drive from all the money you've wasted on gym memberships, still-in-the box exercise machines, and that stash of aerobic and yoga videos in the back of your closet.

Starting Monday assumes that you already know what to eat, recognize the benefits of exercise, and understand what it means to be healthy and take good care of yourself. You've been paying attention all along and get what works. What you haven't figured out yet—and what this book will teach you—is how you can be so smart and still be engaged in such an on-again-off-again relationship with food.

Sadly, the subjects of eating and weight have been treated superficially and simplistically for so many decades— mostly through the promotion of diets—that many people don't realize how humongously complex they actually are. There's the whole biological aspect of appetite and weight, from hormones and brain chemistry to genetic loading and the effects of stress, environmental toxins, and sleep deprivation on appetite. There are the subtle and not-so-subtle messages that food is love, which often come from the profit-driven food industry cooking up and feeding us trash that seduces us into getting hooked on high-fat/salt/sugar cuisine. Additionally, we're barraged by media pressure to diet, diet, diet in order to be thin, thin, thin, which only makes us want to rush out and eat, eat, eat.

This book is about the deeper, less obvious reasons we eat when we don't want to and don't exercise when we do want to. It speaks to the psychological underpinnings of why we don't want to stop overeating, bingeing, and being a couch potato. You already recognize your desire to do better with food, but how far has that knowledge gotten you—to a bookstore or a bakery? Now it's time to learn what keeps you from pursuing and reaching your health and eating goals, which means identifying and coming to terms with the part of you that doesn't want to pursue and reach them. You might be shaking your heads and shouting, "I want my money back for this dumb book because the author is out of her mind. She has no idea how much I desperately want to lose weight/be thin/get healthy." Oh, but I do. I really do. I've walked in your shoes and lived in your skin, but that was long ago.

I've been working with disregulated eaters for more than 30 years, with people who've lost the same bleepin' 50 or 100 pounds over and over, are trapped in the diet-binge cycle, and have at least two or three sizes of clothing in the closet to match their fluctuating weights.

I've written three books on eating (and one for therapists to help them understand and treat disregulated eaters), and have spent half my life teaching the skills of "normal" eating, lecturing across the country, and counseling troubled eaters around the world. I run a message board for emotional eaters and write weekly blogs. Moreover, as I said, I was once a food junkie like you wouldn't believe. In short, I know your eating headaches and heartaches.

The progression of my books for the lay public has not been accidental. My first book, *The Rules of "Normal" Eating*, is a cognitive-behavioral primer on changing food- and weight-related beliefs, feelings and behaviors. *The Food & Feelings Workbook* was written to help emotional eaters follow the rules of appetite by learning to manage their feelings effectively. I also wrote *Nice Girls Finish Fat* to help transform perfectionist-prone, people-pleasing women for whom self-care is done almost exclusively with a fork or spoon.

For decades, I'd wondered about clients' paradoxical behavior—how they could insist they want to be healthy and have a comfortable relationship with food, then go out and overeat to beat the band. As I came to understand more clearly how food-related motivations often waged war against each other, I shared my insights with clients and, lo and behold, they began to have epiphanies about how their desires around food were often mutually exclusive. They began to recognize that their stated intentions—to eat nutritiously, consume food in appropriate portions, get fit, and take good care of themselves—were light years away from their behaviors of bingeing and avoiding regular physical activity.

Identifying and resolving this push-pull tension that kept them stuck in self-abusive patterns made all the difference in treatment and freed them up to make permanent behavioral change. Not swift change, mind you, but the kind that takes your hand and won't let go until it brings you safely to your destination. Realizing that their intent and behavior around food needed to align in order for success to last created in clients a eureka moment—actually dozens of eureka moments. They discovered oddly opposing feelings they never dreamed they had:

- I want to be thin.
  Thin makes me feel vulnerable and scared.

- I can't stand overeating.
  Without food, I'll never feel comforted.

- I should exercise.
  I hate being told I have to do something.

- I deserve to be healthy.
  I'm not worth treating myself lovingly all the time.

Get the picture? Being constantly yanked in two directions, how could these disregulated eaters ever reconcile contradictory beliefs and achieve opposing goals? How could traveling on two divergent paths not make them a little crazy (okay, more than a little)? Once they understood what all the infighting and doing and undoing were all about, they were able to make sense of their seemingly bizarre self-care patterns. Once they realized that all their stops and starts in the eating and exercise arena were not indicative of mental illness but of mental conflict, they could quit beating themselves up and take a more objective look at how to move forward. When they recognized that there was nothing inherently defective about them and that whatever was wrong could be fixed, they began making conscious choices that brought them closer to achieving and sustaining their desired eating and health goals.

Many of you know an encyclopedia's worth of information about eating and weight, but need a dose of self-discovery to identify the mixed feelings that keep you stuck at an eating and self-care impasse. You may have spent years in therapy and read scores of self-help books, but I doubt you've given microscopic and steady scrutiny to your underlying ambivalence. In fact, I know you haven't or you wouldn't be reading this book.

This is good news, folks: You're about to discover new information about your eating problems. You're about to start looking at your relationship with food and your body from the inside out.

In the pages of this book, you'll learn about the seven conflicts that keep you stuck and the keys to unlocking them. You'll discover how to resolve the unconscious dilemmas that have held you back from not merely reaching your goals, but from holding onto your successes.

These seven keys will teach you how to:

1. Create Lasting Change: Stop magical thinking and trying quick fixes and start tolerating discomfort and accepting the hard, incremental work (all done, mind you, in baby steps) it takes to make permanent change with food and your body.

2. Make Conscious Choices: Stop rebelling against "shoulds" and sensible advice about eating and exercise and start making wise choices that are in your long-term best interest.

3. Feel Deserving: Stop believing that you're defective and unfixable and have faith that you deserve to be healthy and fit.

4. Comfort Yourself Effectively: Stop using food for comfort and coping and start practicing life skills for effectively managing stress and distress.

5. Know What's Enough: Stop viewing food and the world through a lens of deprivation and insufficiency and start using a lens of abundance and sufficiency.

6. Manage Intimacy: Stop fearing sexuality and intimacy and start whole-heartedly desiring, seeking, and enjoying closeness.

7. Develop a Healthy Identity: Stop viewing yourself as a sufferer and victim and start seeing yourself as proactive, empowered, and fulfilled.

Every disregulated eater reading this book won't have all of these conflicts. Some might have one or two. Others will find they've cornered the market on mixed feelings. I caution those of you who've had eating struggles throughout your life yet don't relate to any of these conflicts to either reread the list slowly or put it aside for now and come back to it later. The reason is that some folks find it so scary to confront things they don't know about themselves that the doors to their minds slam shut and won't let in any new information. That's okay. Tomorrow can be take-a-peek-at-the-truth day, or the day after. Hopefully, some day soon, your heart and mind will be ready to pry open that door, prop it ajar, and let some fresh ideas blow in.

No one ever said that learning about new aspects of self is fun or easy. But after getting past the ouch of self-recognition, most of us do just fine. And, truth be told, tugging on our hip boots and slogging through our psychological swamps can be exhilarating as well as enlightening.

A few words about the structure of this book. Each of the seven "key" chapters includes "Food for Thought" reflections, a case illustrating the chapter's focus, and homework. In the final chapter, you'll find lists of ideas and practices for pursuing "Further Self-Discovery" relating to each of the seven keys. Incidentally, all clients referred to are composite characters, and their real names are not used.

A reminder of what you won't find in this book: A focus on how to lose weight. My goal here is to guide you along and help you discover whatever is blocking your efforts to sustain "normal" eating and take good care of your health. As you'll see, what you think of as your "eating" problems actually might not be all that much about food. Rather, they might be due to your mixed feelings about yourself and how you interact with the world. So, off we go. From here on, it's all about self-discovery!

CHALLENGES
TO
"NORMAL" EATING

CHAPTER 1

WHY IT'S HARD TO CHANGE OUR EATING

(Help, My Mouth Has a Mind of Its Own!)

D on't you just hate the way we're told what a snap it is to get healthy? Words like "easy, fast, and simple" make you think you can click a switch and, presto, a new, fit "normal" eating you. The truth is that we're fed a constant diet of drivel about how to transform our eating and our bodies, and are convinced our character must be flawed and our motivation sorely lacking if we can't follow a deprivational daily calorie plan for the rest of our lives.

Did you know that the diet industry spends about 60 billion dollars annually to convince us that weight loss plans, products, and programs work?[1] Bombarded with messages trumpeting successful diets and triumphant dieters, we feel like failures. Wrong, wrong, and wrong again! The U.S. has some 72 million dieters, but few enduring success stories.[2]

The diet industry knows that if it can convince us not to trust ourselves around food and get us to believe that we have to be thin to be happy, healthy, and fit, it can keep us hooked going from diet plan to product to program forever. The easier they make it sound, the more likely we are to buy into whatever they're selling.

Studies confirm what our bodies have been telling us all along: diets don't work long term. In fact, 95% of diets fail and most dieters will regain their lost weight in 1-5 years.[3] Tell me, if I offered you an investment opportunity, but warned that your chance of success was five percent, would you whip out your checkbook? I think not. But that's what you've been brainwashed to do when it comes to jumping on the diet bandwagon.

Why can't I just close my eyes and will myself to be a healthy eater?

Before moving on to the premise of this book—that unrecognized fears and mixed feelings can prevent you from reaching and sustaining your eating goals—let me set out what I believe to be true about body weight based on scientific research. In a seminal study on identical and fraternal twins cited in *Rethinking Thin* by *New York Times* science writer Gina Kolata, 70% of the variations in people's weight may be accounted for by inheritance," which is also called genetic loading.[4] In real terms, this statistic is saying that we have *some*, but not *total*, control over the number on the scale. Due to inherited metabolism (more about this in a moment), our weight naturally fluctuates within a range, and it is very hard, if not impossible, to maintain a weight below the lowest point in that range.

So, what *can* we control regarding food and what *is* beyond our ability? Obviously, height and bone structure are pretty well fixed (except with surgery). Metabolism is also more or less set from birth. You may have had a hunch this is true, but who could blame you for shying away from truth in this fat phobic, thin-obsessed culture? We're all unique individuals with differing abilities, temperaments, experiences, and genetics.

> ### *Food for Thought*
>
> Describe your current relationship with food and your body. What have you tried to improve your eating? How has it worked or not worked?

One more point before we move on to the psychological reasons that keep you wrestling with food. Some folks with a host of unhealthy habits *are* able to transform their eating with moderate effort and sustain their new behaviors for life. Here's an example of how that might happen. Let's say a person used to eat only processed, convenience foods, and gave little attention to what and how much she was eating. However, after learning about nutrition and portion monitoring, she became more conscious of mindless eating and began making healthier choices. She could make these changes based on the *educational* part of the word *psychoeducational*: She took new knowledge and was able to run with it without internal conflicts holding her back.

She didn't consider being told to eat nutritiously as a challenge to her autonomy, but was grateful for new information. When she refused sweets and treats, she didn't feel deprived or victimized, but felt proud to be making wiser choices. She didn't feel annoyed at having to plan ahead for her food needs, depressed at cooking for herself, or the urge to use food when she was stressed or distressed.

You and I know painfully well that you are not her. Your reaction to and relationship with food is far more prickly and conflicted. You're not really comfortable in your body whether it's thin or fat, and you can't get food off your mind try as you might. You resist change based on the *psycho* part of the word *psycho-educational*. And, no, in this instance psycho doesn't mean crazy; it's part of the word psycho-logical!

People who succeed at changing their eating habits without a lot of effort do not need to read this book. You do. Most assuredly, they have other problems that you don't. That's life.

Why can't I just say no to food?

Time to face it: There is no quick fix to mending our errant eating ways. That's because eating is an *enormously* complex and complicated subject. Scientists are doing their best to understand how what we eat and weigh are affected by such factors as metabolism, heredity, hormones, stress, exercise, cultural norms, anxiety, addictions, food sensitivities, trauma, sleep, medications, medical problems, and activity level (whew!). If "eating right" were as easy as *just say no*, these folks wouldn't be busting their brains looking for answers.

The science of weight loss is relatively new and there is, of course, a good deal of disagreement about theories and conclusions. Moreover, for every question answered, a slew of new ones arise that demand further study. More proof that the subject of eating and weight is *anything* but simple!

Here are some reasons why:

Metabolism

Metabolism is the process by which we turn food into energy, and it is measured in calories. Technically, a calorie is the quantity of heat necessary to raise by 1° C the temperature of 1 gram of water. The energy produced from calories is what keeps our bodies running and in good repair. Differences in metabolism are due to, among other things, variations in individual physiology that influence how much energy an individual consumes, expends, and stores as fat. These factors are primarily genetically determined but can be altered, to some degree.

Readers of my books know that I teach only the nondiet approach to eating because chronic calorie cutting plays a major role in disregulating our metabolism, sometimes for life. Many of us start dieting in our teens or earlier, and end up eating in ways that can indelibly alter normal biological regulation of appetite and food consumption. Moreover, diets appear to be the gateway activity leading to eating conditions such as anorexia nervosa, bulimia nervosa, and binge eating disorder.

Set Point Theory

One explanation of weight variation is called *set point theory*, which posits that our bodies are preprogrammed genetically to maintain a certain weight and that we can't for long sustain one that is above or below pre-programmed limits. Think of a thermostat with a maximum and minimum setting. Just as a thermostat switches on and off when it hits preset high and low points, so does our body's "fat-o-stat" go on and off. Therefore, if an individual's upper weight limit is, say, 180 pounds, and he consumes more food than is needed to maintain that weight, his body would kick into gear to burn off those extra calories. Similarly, if a person's lower weight limit is 130, and she restricts her food intake so that she's eating less than what would maintain that weight, her metabolism would slow down in order to conserve calories.

Set point is the body's way of making sure that we don't eat too much or too little, but just the right amount to sustain health. Ironically, humans who've survived through the leanest periods of history are the ones who've conserved calories best! For example, in prehistoric times or during famines, if you couldn't pack away and safeguard calories, you'd starve to death, so it was far more advantageous to be heavy (a good calorie conserver) than thin (a mediocre or poor calorie conserver). Remember that set point, cleverly designed through evolution, is not in the least bit interested in whether or not you can get into your bathing suit for that upcoming cruise or how you're going to look at your sister's wedding.

Set point theory is one way of explaining why many people fail to attain or maintain weight goals and why food restriction is often followed by rebound binge eating. In everyday language, when we diet or severely restrict food, our bodies are programmed to react as if food is scarce and work doubly hard to conserve calories, remaining blissfully unaware that we live within walking distance of scads of restaurants and food-marts. Set point theory also explains why people gain back more weight than they originally lost when they stop dieting—their metabolism acts as if another famine (in modern times, another diet) will occur again and builds up extra resources just in case.

What about those people whose metabolisms speed up when they eat too much and keep them slender? They are the anomalies of evolution. Today we consider them fortunate because they seem to be able to eat a great deal and not gain a pound. But that's only because we live in a culture that has an over-abundance of food and hates fat. They'd be the first to go if food were scarce. The good news is that your set point is *not* completely fixed and is influenced by lifestyle choices. So rather than throw up your hands in despair or down a Dove Bar, consider that you may not possess the world's speediest metabolism, but that you have it in your power to increase its effectiveness through food choice and exercise and other lifestyle choices such as managing stress better and getting enough sleep.

Body Structure and Type

Although we often use fashion to accentuate the positive and de-accentuate the negative according to cultural norms and what body type is in vogue, short of surgery, we can't change the basic structure of our bodies. It's tragic that we don't live in a society that values all shapes and sizes. Those of us who don't have the culturally-ideal body type have two choices: we either spend our lives lamenting this fact or work on accepting what we can't change. We can't choose our body structure, but we sure as heck can determine our attitude about it. Enough said.

Appetite Regulation

Ever wonder exactly how appetite works? What makes us hungry? What makes us full? We are highly efficient machines, and appetite regulation operates on the principle of fuel in and energy out. Through brain chemicals that process the body's energy and fuel needs, the body signals us to eat, and when we have enough potential energy stored as fat, it sends out a message to stop eating. Pretty clever, huh?

Without getting too scientific, an appetite stimulant called ghrelin is released when the hypothalamus senses that the body is low on energy. Along with ghrelin, insulin regulates hunger levels, and leptin produces feelings of satiation and suppression of appetite to make us want to stop eating. Insulin is also involved with fat storage.

The amount and proportion of chemicals in our bodies involved with appetite are passed down (for better or worse) from our parents. If you never feel full or satiated, it's possible that you're someone with a hormonal imbalance, which can be identified through laboratory testing. Along with appetite regulators, heredity also passes along genes that influence what we weigh. Of note are gene mutations, which correlate to obesity because of how they promote increased fat storage. For more information on the intricacies of appetite, I recommend the highly informative, myth busting *Health at Every Size: The Surprising Truth about Your Weight* by Linda Bacon, Ph.D.

Neurotransmitters

People who take antidepressant or anti-anxiety medications know something about neurotransmitters. They're the brain chemicals responsible for our moods and for "mood disorders." Neurotransmitters are brain chemicals that modulate electrical signals between neurons and other cells, biochemical agents that transmit information from one cell to another to regulate mood and affect. They're the brain's chemical messengers that make us feel up or down, blue and blah, upbeat and euphoric, calm or excited, anxious or panicky. Commonly known neurotransmitters include serotonin and gamma-aminobutyric acid (GABA) which soothe and relax us when we're upset, dopamine which generates that buzz of euphoria, and norepinephrine which keeps us focused and alert.

> ## Food for Thought
>
> Which of the previous factors might influence your inability to eat "normally"—metabolism, genetics, neurotransmitter imbalances? Give examples.

Can a neurotransmitter imbalance cause me to engage in unwanted eating?

Because many disregulated eaters tend to turn to food when they're stressed or distressed, you might think that neurotransmitters have something to do with when and what you eat—and you'd be right! We crave carbohydrates when we're stressed because, in the short term (*only*), they make us feel better. They do this because these foods are made up of substances which interact with brain chemicals to affect our mood.

You know how heavenly it feels when you're eating a yummy muffin top or a plate of *fettuccini Alfredo?* That's because the ingredients in these foods generate bursts of dopamine, the "feel good" neurotransmitter. Why these foods as opposed to, say, spinach or tuna fish? Because muffins and pasta are made up of sugar and fat, the exact energy sources we need to keep us going when food is scarce. Through evolution, we're primed to seek foods high in sugar and fat, which will sustain us better than protein. That delightful surge of dopamine ensures that we'll return to this same food source again and again. When folks talk about having a food "orgasm," they're not far from wrong. It makes sense that we're programmed by blasts of feel-good chemicals to do the two things humans must do to survive as a species: eat and make babies.

Moreover, due to genetic loading or stressful childhoods (or, more likely, a combination of both), we often end up with an ineffective complement of neurotransmitters. Lacking sufficient serotonin or GABA, we may have a hard time regulating our moods, because there's not enough available to soothe us. Can you see where this line of thinking is going? When we're deficient in internal relaxers, it makes total sense to turn to foods that break down into chemicals which affect the brain—and make us feel better. Unfortunately, these are the same goodies that are high in sugar and fat.

Food Addictions and Allergies

The jury is out on whether or not sugar is technically addictive: some studies say yes and others say no. If you've had food problems for ages, you probably feel addicted to sugar. By eating it regularly, craving increases but, take a break for a while, and you may lose your desire for it. Assuming that sugar could well be addictive, it's logical that some people will become dependent on it and some will not. Just as there are folks who can drink alcohol or even use heroin without craving these substances physiologically, most people can consume sweets and not develop a sugar jones. However, it makes sense that people with a chemical imbalance will seek foods to bliss themselves out and continue to crave them.

Allergies are bona fide physical conditions that cause bodily discomfort, and can be confirmed through medical testing. The most common food allergies are to wheat (gluten), eggs, dairy, soy, shellfish, and peanuts. In an authentic food allergy, the immune system makes the error of identifying a food as harmful, which generates the production of antibodies to fight this alleged enemy. People with food allergies can have mild to life-threatening symptoms—hives, welts, swelling, breathing problems, nausea, diarrhea or abdominal pain, dizziness or fainting—which usually arise within an hour of eating the offending food. Less threatening are food intolerances and sensitivities, which often cause abdominal pain or bloating in response to consuming the foods listed above.

There are two reasons I bring up this subject. One is that many disregulated eaters have true food allergies, which make it even more difficult for them to make healthy, satisfying food choices. On top of having to consider food content such as fiber, protein, fat and sugar, they need to be on the lookout for soy, dairy, eggs or gluten. This makes life very difficult indeed, but with the right mindset is eminently doable. The second reason is that many troubled eaters say that food allergies are causing their eating problems when they don't know this for a fact. I'm all for intuition and learning from experience, but when it comes to identifying allergies, your best bet is to be tested for them.

The Food Industry

There's no way to have a serious discussion of factors affecting eating and weight without mentioning what has happened within the food industry over the last century. Grabbing a top market share, extending product shelf-life, getting kids hooked on sugar and fat early on, and making it appear that quick-and-easy dishes are better for you and your family than real food that takes longer to prepare are just some ways the food industry does not have society's best interest at heart. Their bottom line is profit and yours is health, and any fool can see how these end goals are mutually exclusive.

The food industry has shaped our eating preferences and, through them, even may be changing our brains. According to Dr. Linda Bacon, Ph.D., "Some animal studies suggest that repeated and frequent exposure to fatty foods reconfigures the brain to crave still more fat."[5] And who do you think is behind the push for eating more fatty, salty, sugary, and processed foods? The food industry, of course. For a fascinating and fact-based critique of our food manufacturers, read *The End of Overeating: Taking Control of the Insatiable American Appetite* by David A. Kessler, MD.

Is there any hope for me?

Enough social and scientific commentary. Let's talk about you and *your* eating troubles. My guess is that you fall into one of two categories: 1) You've been struggling to eat more healthily for ages with little or no success, or 2) You've had times of healthy or "normal" eating which ended abruptly or slipped away gradually. In this second case, after every frustrating and unsuccessful attempt to "control" your appetite through diet or food restriction, you've beaten yourself up for your perceived failures and returned to dreaming of eating "normally" the way other people dream of winning the lottery. Now you avoid mirrors, are disconnected from and possibly disgusted with your body, and can't believe you're reading yet another book to try to make peace with food!

What I want to impress upon you is that you have yet to make permanent peace with food because different parts of your mind have been at war with each other. You've been held back by forces that in some ways have everything to do with eating and health and in some ways have nothing to do with it. Your underlying conflicts would be playing out (and may, in fact, *be* playing out) in other arenas if you didn't have eating problems. These are psychological, not eating, issues.

And this is exactly why there *is* hope for you. Think of what you're about to learn as, trite as it sounds, fixing the foundation of your house. All these years, you've been patching the walls and ceilings and redecorating. Now you're going down to the basement to make sure that the foundation is solid and won't keep shifting underneath you.

You're embarking on a journey to heal the internal mixed feelings that have been driving your unhealthy relationship with food and your body for decades. By discovering what kinds of conflicted thinking produce your contradictory behaviors around food, exercise and self-care, you'll be removing the obstacles to enjoying a lifetime of health and wellness.

Food for Thought

What are the current barriers that prevent you from improving your eating? What do you need to tell yourself to achieve success?

HOMEWORK:

Write out these answers for yourself.

1. From the factors listed, which do you think impact your eating and weight?

2. What factors had you not considered before?

3. Which new concepts or ideas about the complexity of eating and weight made you feel better or more hopeful?

4. Which thoughts about the complexity of eating and weight made you feel uncomfortable or anxious?

5. Based on this chapter, what changes in your thinking and understanding about the complexities of food and weight will make it easier to move forward in a positive, healthy direction?

---

[1] *U.S. Weight Loss Market Worth $60.9 Billion, http://www.prweb.com/releases/2011/5/prweb8393658.htm,* retrieved 6/5/13

[2] *http://fatfacts.pbworks.com/w/page/6734330/Dieting%20Statistics,* retrieved 6/5/13

[3] *Statistics on Weight Discrimination: A Waste of Talent,* Council on Size and Weight Discrimination, www.cswd.org, retrieved 6/5/13.

[4] Kolata, G. (2007), *Rethinking Thin,* New York: Picador, page 123.

[5] Bacon, L. (2008), *Health at Every Size: The Surprising Truth About Your Weight,* Dallas, TX: Benbella Books.

CHAPTER 2

REASONS WE WANT TO EAT "NORMALLY"

(Stop Me When I Get to Infinity!)

Y ou might be thinking, *Why on earth* wouldn't *I want to eat "normally" and take care of my health?* Of course, you want to stop obsessing about every morsel you put into your mouth and really savor the exquisite delight food can bring. I bet you've never given a moment's thought to the fact that you could possibly want anything *but* a positive relationship with food and your body.

Frankly, it's nearly impossible not to be hyper-focused on weight these days, living as we do in the most fat-phobic, thin-obsessed culture in the history of the world. We're told day in and day out that our eating habits are unacceptable, our bodies substandard, and we will never be happy unless we weigh less. This all adds up to convincing us that what's important about us is on the outside not on the inside. No matter how utterly amazing we are, the final judgment is that we should not and will not be okay until we reach a totally arbitrary body ideal.

Sadly, an acceptable standard of thinness is unlikely to be achieved by most of us and dreaming the impossible dream only shreds our mental health and self-esteem. Even healthy, average weight people often think—erroneously—that they need to shed pounds. We're bombarded daily with information that says we're unfit, fat and flabby even when we're not, and too often walk around feeling guilty for not being thinner and fitter. Undoubtedly, most of you who are reading this book have been struggling for years with food, but it pays to stop and consider whether you're chasing an impossible weight loss ideal—and in the process creating eating problems for yourself. What I'm saying here is if it ain't broke, don't fix it.

This chapter describes common reasons for wanting to eat well and care for your body, but in order to understand your motivation more fully, you will need to identify your own reasons for wishing to achieve these goals.

Food for Thought

Right now, in order of priority, what are *your* top three reasons for wanting to become a "normal" eater?

Isn't "Thou shalt be thin" the 11th Commandment?

Now that you've identified your primary motivations for wanting to improve your relationship with food, let's see what other possibilities are floating around. Alternate reasons don't make yours wrong. Read them with curiosity and without judgment, and consider each one as a potential motivator. Be honest. This book is about exploring and discovering *new* information about what food, eating, and body size mean to *you*!

Reasons for Wanting to be a "Normal" Eater

REASON: To meet a cultural ideal

You've already heard my rant about how obsessed society is with eating and weight. This puts us in the position of constantly measuring ourselves against an unrealistic ideal that most of us will never come near to achieving. We've been brainwashed into believing that if we are thin, all our problems will disappear. Whether you realize it or not, the subtext of many media messages is that the good life will be ours if we'd only wise up about slimming down.

Every time we gaze at beanstalk magazine models and digitally-enhanced celebrities, we are reminded of what we are not—thin enough. Although all around us there are folks as fat as or fatter than we are, we still are left with the impression that the smart and successful ones have whittled themselves down to svelte while we failures just can't seem to get—or stay—with the program. I have clients who swear they never see people as overweight as they are and that there are no heavy people on the planet having fun. To prove them wrong, I keep a wedding announcement photo of a plus-size couple within reach in therapy sessions to whip out and give clients a dose of reality

What this hyper focus on thinness does is to negate all the good things we have going for us—warm and generous hearts, creativity, topnotch brains, integrity, passion—and replace them with, well, nothing meaningful. No matter how successful we are, if we haven't met society's body size standards, we too often come to believe that we're worth zilch.

I once had a client, a teacher, come to see me in tears the week before she was about to receive a highly coveted local award for which she'd worked long and hard. Care to guess why she was upset? Because all she could think about (other than her acceptance speech) was that people would see a fat woman at the podium and forget about all her achievements. How sad is that?

Which brings me to the point that too many of us put how we look ahead of who we are. I heard a heartbreaking anecdote from a friend who attended a pricey fundraising dinner and had a chance to hob knob with some prominent national and international figures, household names for many of us, including a well-known dignitary we'll call Madame X. On the receiving line at the end of the event, my friend asked her to sign a photograph of them together taken at a similar event decades before. And, what do you think Madame X had to say? After signing the photo, she shook her head in dismay and lamented that she'd been so much thinner back then!

We really have some twisted thinking about weight. Sometimes we go so far as to project *our* thoughts into *other* people's heads and believe that they're disgusted with our fatness (because we are), but that they'd admire and envy us if we were thinner. We think we're two thumbs down at our present weight and will automatically become two thumbs up by dropping inches or pounds. We're so consumed with this kind of craziness that we totally lose sight of who we are and our value as human beings.

If you're morbidly obese, it's understandable that you desire to look "normal," and that getting to a more average weight may actually change people's perception of you. Even so, be careful to avoid getting seduced into believing that weight reduction will make your fantasies come true. For people who feel a need to lose 30 pounds or less, the fact is that imagining that life will suddenly be a bed of roses when you "get there" is patently untrue. It's time to shatter the myth that happiness is one or five sizes smaller than you are now. There are thin people who are miserable and fat people who exude joy and purpose. Weight is only one factor among many that impacts whether and how you reach your potential.

Food for Thought

How influenced are you by weight and beauty standards? In concrete terms, what will change if you get thinner? What will stay the same? What do you imagine will happen if you switch your focus from losing weight to eating "normally"?

REASON: *To gain approval from family*

Now we're moving from the impersonal—culture—to the personal—those influential and often judgmental people in your life: your family members. It makes sense that you want to be accepted by those who are close to you. However, it can be pathologically unhealthy to go overboard seeking approval from them. Most people want to be attractive or, at the least, presentable. It tickles us to hear compliments and we enjoy brief rushes from looking our best, but that's about as far as it should go.

Too many folks believe they'll only be loved or accepted once they've lost enough weight. Unfortunately, this belief goes beyond appearance and generally stems from how little unconditional love they received as children. Kids need and deserve unqualified love to thrive. They must know that they can make mistakes and utterly fail, be wrong, inappropriate, and march to their own drums, and that parental love will still be there for them. That doesn't mean that parents and adults have to ignore or excuse bad behavior. It does mean that children need to feel cherished and adored in spite of their faults, and that adults must be convinced beyond a shadow of a doubt that they are basically lovable no matter what they look like.

Too few of us grew up experiencing unconditional love. Individuals who end up as people-pleasers were shaped by a particular dynamic set up in their families. Please Mom or Dad (even if it meant displeasing or denying yourself) and you were showered with smiles and hugs (and maybe a few material possessions to boot). Displease your parents (because you were trying to honor your own desires) and you were ignored, demeaned, invalidated, rejected, marginalized, shamed, or punished. As children, we are totally dependent on our parents and will do anything and everything to please them because the idea of being abandoned (physically or emotionally) by them is too terrible to contemplate. It's instinct: we do what we have to do to—we adapt—to survive.

If parents encourage us to make age-appropriate decisions rather than impose their will or viewpoint on us, our own opinions come to mean more and more to us as we mature and, as adults, our parents' judgments are far less important than our own. Good mental health means following our own hearts and giving ourselves final approval! However, if parents undermine our early choices and silence our childhood voices, we become scared to think for ourselves (especially to think well of ourselves) and excessively depend on others' opinions.

Please understand that I'm not speaking only of appearance-related issues. I'm talking about the basic way your parents and other adults encouraged or discouraged you from deciding what was right and wrong *for you*. Maybe they never said a word about eating or weight, but made it painfully clear that you couldn't possibly know what's best for you and should listen only to them in order to be happy and successful. Maybe the unspoken message—which came across loud and clear—was my-way-or-the-highway. Maybe they so feared your making mistakes that they discouraged you from learning by trial and error.

Here's an example of what I mean. A few years ago I was chatting with the daughter of an acquaintance who had just graduated from college with a degree in astrophysics. I congratulated her and said she must be tremendously proud of herself. Expecting her to agree, I was taken aback when she smiled nervously and said that she hoped her parents were proud of her. Ever the therapist, I told her that it was important at her age to feel proud of her achievement and that it would, of course, be icing on the cake if her parents were proud of her too. Honestly, she looked at me blankly, as if she didn't understand a word I was saying or couldn't conceive of anything being more important than pleasing her parents. Sadly, she reminded me of many of my clients.

Obviously, if Dad teased you about your love handles and Mom frowned at those extra portions you heaped on your plate, a desire to avoid their judgment may make you unsure of how you should eat today. If you were given the message that there was something awry with your appetite or defective about your body, you probably began to believe that you can't trust your own food choices and, instead, are focused on what others believe is right for you.

By obsessing about eating and weight, you may not realize that what you're really seeking is Mom or Dad's love and approval. Whether you're 19 or 39 or 79, or if your parents are alive or dead, this dynamic may be at work. Or perhaps you were competitive with siblings, vying for parental attention, and still want to outshine them to win Mom or Dad's applause. Now, as a grownup, if you're still questing for your parents' love *for any reason whatsoever*, you have not fully emotionally matured. For a healthy adult, it's gravy when parents value and approve of who you are and what you do, but it's unessential and relatively inconsequential if they don't. If your parents can't love you for exactly who you are, that's *their* problem, not *yours*. How sad for them and for you, but time's a wastin' and you have to move on. This is a difficult process and takes working through a great many painful, grief-filled feelings. A place to start is not seeking their approval for your eating, weight, or appearance.

I recall a client who at age 40 was terribly enmeshed with her parents with whom she lived, an enmeshment which had grown stronger after her sister died from complications of anorexia nervosa. My client would be on her way out of the house and her mother would stop her halfway through the doorway to button up her sweater! And my client let her. She couldn't bear to see her mother upset, which involved a torrent of tears and other histrionics, and therefore, lived to make her happy. Because her father was physically abusive, she also tiptoed around him. At one point, she married a nice man, but her parents undermined the marriage and my client eventually divorced her husband and returned home.

She also had to be hospitalized several times for anorexia, yet her parents actually discouraged her from "normal" eating. Sadly, they feared that if she became healthy, she would move out and leave them alone in their marital misery. They needn't have worried. By the time she was an adult, she was so dependent on their telling her what was right and wrong that she believed she could never figure it out on her own. I offer this extreme example to show the lengths that adult children will go to seek parental love.

Similarly, if you're used to diets telling you what to eat and not eat, you probably have given up trusting yourself and desperately yearn for external direction and reinforcement. You live for the encouragement of those Weight Watchers, OA, or Jenny Craig cheerleaders and for the admiration of fellow program members when you drop a few pounds. However, a word of caution: The more you seek their approval—any outside approval—the less you will rely on valuing your own. Building self-trust and self-validation is key to sustaining healthy behaviors for life.

Food for Thought

Be honest. Would your Mom or Dad love or approve of you more if you were thinner? What toll does trying to win their praise take on you? What will happen if you stop seeking their approval on eating and weight? On other things?

REASON: To improve health and fitness

In fact, wanting to improve health and fitness are two of the best reasons you could have for reading this book: they're clear and straightforward and based on moving toward positive goals. Compare them to the desire to have a perfect body based on cultural standards or to attain the unwinnable love of emotionally stunted parents.

However, one risk with pursuing health and fitness goals is that you may become too rigid about food or excessive about exercise. If people get too gung ho starting nutritious food plans and exercise programs, their enthusiasm and commitment may wane shortly thereafter. Also, you don't want your major focus to be on food and fitness. You want to have a full and satisfying life. Unless you're a competitive athlete, it's best to avoid questions about what and when to eat and how long to spend at the gym. If you're not in training, your life should be brimming with varied interests, passions, and pursuits.

Food for Thought

Why are you interested in improving your relationship with food? Is your major focus on healthy eating? What exactly are your fitness goals? Is activity for you about weight loss or health gain? How do you see fitness and "normal" eating fitting into your larger self-care goals?

REASON: To get a date or keep a mate

This is another one of those not-so-great reasons to eat better with the hopes of losing weight. Can you guess why? Like trying to gain approval from parents, improving your eating to lose weight for someone else is a self-defeating exercise in external approval-seeking. All your energies be-come funneled into what she'll think or what he'll say. Or you engage in endless fantasies about how sexy and seduc-tive you'll be with your new body and miss out on the pre-sent moment.

What happens if you had a great week with food and feel proud of yourself, but don't get the praise you'd hoped for from your date or partner—or any notice at all? What happens to how your carry yourself and approach potential partners when you assume they won't be romantically inter-ested in you at your size? What kind of self-esteem are you building when you put more attention on what others think of you than on what you think of yourself?

Let's take one scenario at a time. First, getting a date. This assumes that you want one. Some people are fine (re-ally fine, I swear) living a life without a romantic interest. Life is replete and satisfying with work, connections, friends, passions, and any other darned thing they want to fill it up with. So, start by asking yourself if you truly want to date or find a mate or only think you should. Maybe you do and maybe you don't; either way is fine as long as you're speak-ing authentically from your heart.

Okay, let's assume you yearn to find someone special and permanent. It's true that because of cultural fat phobia, some prospects may make superficial judgments about how you look. You know it and I know it and, sad as this fact is, that's life. However, let's not fall into an all-or-nothing trap here. Not everyone is thin-obsessed. There are loving couples out there in every shape and size. Hello, look around. Then again, maybe there's some hypocrisy going on and maybe you have weight prejudices of your own when it comes to potential partners.

As an aside, there are many physical traits that turn potential lovers on or off. I know a thin woman who went on a blind date and at the end of it, he told her he couldn't abide her seriously curly hair. At five feet, I've had men tell me they don't care for petite women because we seem so fragile. Moreover, at my height, I've never been attracted to short men, but preferred taller guys. Go figure.

Years ago I had a client who was 250 pounds and dated frequently, but she always felt she couldn't be choosy and had to accept whoever came along. She decided that she'd stop dating and start again when she lost 100 pounds, but when she reached 170, she said the heck with it and began putting herself out into the dating scene. Once again, she had a good number of men interested in her, but no one she was eager to date. She continued to shed pounds over time and eventually reached 150 pounds, but was still dismayed that she couldn't attract the kind of guy she wanted. Through therapy she finally realized that it wasn't her weight that was keeping her from finding Mr. Right, but the fact that she'd had an emotionally abusive father and a passive, martyr of a mother and *that* was the kind of relationship that felt familiar to her. Once she learned to read potential partners' red flags better, she was able to find emotionally healthier men more to her liking.

I also knew a beautiful, plus-size woman who had a flair for fashion and was active and involved in her community. Shortly after her wedding, I happened to be in a meeting where she was passing around her bridal photos. I loved it: she was in a bright red dress and was one of the most beautiful brides I'd ever seen. She would have laughed if you'd told her that no one would be interested in her at her size or that she should have worn a dress that didn't call attention to her body. Self-esteem works from the inside out, not the outside in.

What I've come to realize from my decades of treating people who are average weight, obese, or have anorexia sounds corny, but I believe it is 100% true: people who feel ugly inside, feel ugly outside. Thinness, beauty, and having an ideal body are merely symbols of wanting something else, just as food when you're not hungry represents some other craving. Of course, being closer to a norm makes life easier for *some* people, but over-focusing on appearance for a lifetime simply wears a person down.

Food for Thought

Do you feel that no one will be interested in or love you at your current size? On what do you base your opinion? What, other than losing weight, could prompt you to put yourself out on the dating scene?

Now, let's move on to the second issue, keeping a mate. It can be tough for partners who've married someone slim or of average weight to watch as their partner puts on pounds. This is not a matter of right versus wrong. We are physically attracted to people for certain reasons and, as we age, that attraction often continues—though sometimes it disappears for varying reasons. For many couples, when one partner gains a lot of weight, their relationship stays passionate and loving. However, if things are already sliding downhill or if there isn't much holding a couple together to begin with other than physical attraction (which is more often the case when people marry young or on the rebound), there's a chance that weight gain will become the focus of unhappiness.

When a partner dislikes her (or his) looks or weight, she might also have an aversion to being touched or seen naked. Desire is squelched and physical intimacy becomes taboo. As she withdraws, body size gets the blame when what's holding her back is often emotional or physical discomfort. Communication stops, intimacy and sex vanish, and partners drift apart. The only way to get back on track is to talk about what's going on—and what's not!

If you're someone whose partner overtly states or covertly implies that she will only love you thin or if you lose weight, you're in a tough situation. Although it may be the truth—maybe your mate is incapable of loving you as is—it's hard not to feel rotten about yourself and angry at your partner. What if you lose the weight and she still doesn't want you, because your relationship problems go far deeper than just your size or shape?

Food for Thought

Are you in a relationship in which your spouse or partner is unhappy with your weight or the shape you're in? How is this expressed? How does this make you feel and act? Have you calmly and lovingly shared the effect his or her comments have on you?

REASON: To feel more comfortable in your body

This is another excellent reason to work on developing "normal" eating skills. So many disregulated eaters talk about not feeling like themselves when they're carrying around more weight than they'd like. They think of them-selves as having a thin or average body, and are shocked when they look in the mirror and find a large individual staring back at them. Be aware that being comfortable in your body isn't about just shedding pounds. Folks who reg-ularly overeat often disconnect from body sensations and cues in other ways, as well. Even though disregulated eaters, including undereaters, may believe they're thinking about their bodies 24/7, they too often have severed connection to appetite and physical signals of pleasure and pain, and are not really *in* their bodies most of the time, certainly not when they eat. Often they're mentally in the body they used to have or the one they wish or hope to have some day. As one of my clients says, "It's as if I'm only connected with what's going on in my head. The rest of my body is just *there* carrying my head around."

People who are uncomfortable in their bodies often ig-nore or don't register signs of discomfort. Moreover, they rarely enjoy physical pleasure (other than the pain-tinged frenzy of eating) because they believe they don't deserve joy and good feelings. As weight piles on, they engage in de-creased physical activity, avoid being touched, and decrease self-care in general. They might as well be walking around with a visible head and no body at all. The goal is not only to become comfortable in your body, but to feel totally con-nected to and loving toward it.

Sometimes plus-size folks start to make these connec-tions through gentle exercise, dance, yoga, or massage. I en-courage clients to keep looking at their bodies until their reaction is neutral and non-judgmental. This can take a long time and gobs of self-compassion. Usually they flinch at first glance and look away from the mirror, but gradually they're able to reduce judgment and identify parts of their bodies they admire. When they begin to reconnect to themselves physically, they often start to become more active which also generates increased body connection, creating a positive, rather than a negative, feedback loop.

The desire to be comfortable in your body in order to engage in activities is a fabulous reason to eat more "normally" and get fit. Desiring to be comfortable in your body is a healthy reason to improve your eating, especially because your motivation is pleasing yourself not someone else. *You* do the work and *you* get the benefits.

Food for Thought

How comfortable are you in your body? Other than losing weight, what would make you more comfortable? What makes you less comfortable? What activities have you given up because of your weight? Which ones would you like to engage in if you were more fit? Which ones could you engage in at your current fitness level and size?

REASON: *To be in charge of eating and your body*

One of our natural instincts is the drive to be in charge of ourselves and our environment. It makes sense that the more power and autonomy we have, the safer and more secure we feel. When I talk about being in charge of eating and body, I certainly do not mean dictatorial control, but, rather, caring for yourself in a wise, gentle, loving, and compassionate manner—knowing what's best for you, taking good care of yourself, and acting in ways that enhance your quality of life and are in your long-term self-interest.

For too many years when it comes to eating, we've talked about "control," a term which smacks of pressure, restriction, and holding on tight. But saying "no" is only half the equation, and the reason that control never works to help us eat "normally." Sure, it's vital to know when to move away from food, but it's equally important to recognize when to say yes and move toward it. To be in charge is to be skilled in self-regulation—sensing both a need for more and a need for less in whatever you're doing, including eating—which is an excellent goal, rather than one of self-control.

Self-regulation is essential in managing nearly every aspect of life. Without a keen ability to respond appropriately around food, you either eat rigidly and restrictively (exerting control), overeat and binge-eat (give up control), or yo-yo back and forth between the two. If your goal is to effectively regulate your eating to stop obsessing about weight and enjoy food for nourishment and pleasure, three cheers for you. By paying attention to appetite cues and body connections, you'll make wiser decisions, self-trust will grow, and you'll feel in better balance.

Desiring to be in charge of eating and your body means being ready to act more wisely and take self-care more seriously. This means shifting your attention away from obsessing about weight, and moving on with life. It involves casting your net wide—beyond your pantry—to find your passions and pleasures. Taking charge of your eating is the first step in taking charge of your life!

Food for Thought

How does lack of self-regulation with food affect your life? How does it affect your self-perception? How would it feel to be more adept at regulating your eating? What other parts of your life would you like to be in charge of and regulate more effectively?

So, there you have it: the major reasons most folks want to eat "normally." Maybe these reasons are nothing new to you. Big deal, you might be thinking, I knew all that. If so, excellent! What I'm trying to illustrate in this chapter is the recognition that there are both more and less *effective* motivations to change eating habits. For example, wanting to eat better to lose weight or for someone else's approval are not as effective motivators as doing so to be in charge of your eating or to feel more comfortable in your body. Moreover, by helping you identify both general incentives and your particular ones for wanting a better relationship with food, I'm laying the groundwork for further understanding that there also may be a hidden set of motivators that *keep* you from reaching your eating and health goals. If you're game for discovering what they are, read on.

HOMEWORK

Write out these answers for yourself.

1. What did you learn in this chapter about your motivation to be a "normal" eater?

2. What motivations for "normal" eating were new to you?

3. Which new concepts or ideas made you feel better or more hopeful?

4. Which new concepts or ideas made you feel uncomfortable or anxious?

5. Based on this chapter, what can you do to ensure that your motivation to eat "normally" will be most effective in the long-term?

CHAPTER 3

HOW INTERNAL CONFLICTS PREVENT US FROM EATING "NORMALLY"

(In This Corner We Have Me and in This Corner We Have—Me!)

In this chapter, you'll learn first about how the mind works in general and, second, how your mind may be derailing you from reaching *your* eating goals. You'll never resolve your eating struggles without understanding the nature and purpose of mixed feelings and why so much of what we believe and feel resides woefully outside of our awareness. After this chapter, it's on to the seven keys, so tune into the general psychology channel for now knowing we'll be switching to your very oen self-discovery channel in just a bit.

Isn't "unconscious" what happens when you fall on your head?

Even in our modern world, mention the word "unconscious" and some people's eyes glaze over and they start shaking their heads as if someone's talking about voodoo or alien abduction. Rather than go into a lengthy clinical explanation of what we call the unconscious, simply think of it as aspects of self of which you are unaware or only partially aware. There is no actual part of the brain that is a receptacle for these perceptions. In fact, the unconscious is not a thing at all—not a tidy, little bin with a sign tacked on saying " Unknown Information, Forgotten Memories, and Things That Make Me Uncomfortable"—but a theoretical construct. Think of it as a process or mechanism rather than as a storage site.

In 1955 Joseph Luft and Harrington Ingham developed a schematic model called the Johari Window that is helpful in understanding the concept of the unconscious process.[1]

DIAGRAM OF JOHARI WINDOW

	KNOWN BY SELF	UNKNOWN BY SELF
KNOWN BY OTHERS	*Open/free area or arena*	*Blind area or blind spot*
UNKNOWN BY OTHERS	*Hidden area or façade*	*Unknown area*

The "open/free *arena*" quadrant includes what's known by you and about you by others. It contains all the reasons you recognize for wanting to eat well that others also know about you—such as your desire to be healthy. This is information that you share with others.

The information in your "hidden or *façade*" area is also known to you, but is not known to others. These are our secrets. For instance, even your intimates may not know that you have a huge crush on a subordinate and are anxious about him judging you as you eat lunch together.

To understand unconscious motivation, we're most interested in the next two quadrants: *blind spots* and *unknown* areas. Blind spots are just that— things others see about us that we can't. They include truths that we've never considered and, hence, of which we're totally ignorant, as well as nuggets of truth that we may have an inkling about but would rather not openly acknowledge. Think of blind spots this way: Just because you lack awareness of particular characteristics about yourself, doesn't mean they're not abundantly clear to others. For example, you may fail to recognize that you're a bit stingy tipping at restaurants and that this is why your friends always offer to figure out the tip for you.

The *unknown* arena is composed of self-truths of which you and others are unaware. Not that these self parts or snippets of information don't exist. They do, only they're buried deep. Perhaps you have a friend who eats only organic foods and is obsessed with avoiding sugar and flour. His quest to maintain good health may be driven by a hidden fear of dying young, like his father, although he's never made this mental connection and neither have you.

Fortunately, where information falls on the conscious/unconscious continuum or within the quadrants of the Johari Window is anything but fixed. Blind area information may gradually or suddenly spring into awareness. For example, referring to the above examples, at some point you may sheepishly admit the truth of your stinginess and decide to become a more generous tipper, and your vegan friend may recognize that he's terrified of dying prematurely. Most of us have what we think of as brief, unexpected "ah ha" moments in which new information bursts into awareness and brings what we think or do into clarity.

> ### Food for Thought
>
> How comfortable are you with the concept of not knowing things about yourself? About others knowing things about you that you don't? Would you say you're generally aware or unaware of how you think, feel and act? What would help you become more aware?

Okay, enough with the psychology lesson. My point is that there are aspects of self that remain under our radar, not necessarily permanently, but locked away until we go searching for them or accidentally stumble upon them. If you've ever tried to point out someone's shortcomings and they seem to have no clue what you're talking about—when it's obvious to the immediate world and then some—you know exactly what I mean. They can't see what they can't see. The desire to remain ignorant is an integral but frustrating part of human nature.

Obviously, no one can be totally aware of themselves all the time. On the other hand, sleepwalking through life is not recommended. There are too many sharp objects to bump into. The goal of human potential is to live as consciously as possible while recognizing and accepting that we all have limits to what we know about ourselves, a tricky balance. This dynamic is called a *paradox*, a knowing that there's stuff we don't know. Ironically, some folks spend their entire lives chasing down self-knowledge and are severely disappointed that they never fully capture it all, while others flee from the most evident self truths as if knowing them will cause them to self-destruct on the spot.

What gives the unconscious such a bad rap?

Now that you understand the basic concepts of consciousness (in awareness) and unconsciousness (outside of awareness), it's time to take a look at what kind of information falls into each category. Generally, conscious material has the following gate-keeper characteristics:

Conscious material is **familiar** and provides **security.**

We don't think much about what's familiar because we take it for granted as truth. Familiar information is stuff we've learned since we can remember (and even before that)—our heritage, personality traits, gender roles, etc. There's comfort in telling yourself, "Yeah, that's me, always trying to befriend someone and getting hurt in the process" or "I'm shy." Whether or not these assessments happen to be true is beside the point; we become attached to perceptions that are familiar to us, be they positive or negative. They may make us happy or unhappy, but nevertheless they breed a certain security-blanket reassurance because they help us believe that we know ourselves, thereby giving us more control over life than we actually have.

Many disregulated eaters—many people, in general—

are adamant about their belief in who they are. They're *never* this or they're *always* that. I once had to ban a client from using the words "always" and "never" in our sessions because she could barely get through a sentence without them. Eventually I asked why those words seemed so necessary to her, and she replied that saying them aloud helped her sort out the inner confusion she'd had about herself since childhood, based on her father needing to be right and insisting that she had no idea what she thought or felt. As she matured, she wrapped herself in the security of words, as if to say, "This *is* who I am. I *do* know what I think and feel."

On a personal note, for years I used to tell myself that I'm no good at technical matters. I'd get a lump in my throat and a tightness in my chest every time I went to pry open a box that contained any sort of technology and had to read instructions that had more than three steps. One day, my friend and I were about to set up a new digital gadget and, rather than let her take the lead as I usually did (because I considered *her* tech savvy), I impatiently pulled out the instructions and got to work. When the job was complete, my friend commented on how well I'd done (and she didn't sound surprised either). So, I've revised my persona to that of a person who is as technically skilled as the next person. And, you know what, I'm now the go-to person in my house when a machine breaks down or a new one needs setting up!

Conscious material is **superficial** and easily **accessed.**

Too many of us don't like to dig deep to find out what we're feeling or thinking. We hate to "dwell," hate to reach, preferring what's out there for the taking, the low-hanging fruit we can easily pluck off the tree of self-knowledge. We look around and see that other people appear content doing what we're doing and, hence, assume we should be content too—you know, like, diets are fun and thinness is the key to happiness. So, we don't think too hard about how we're feeling and, instead, make assumptions about our emotions. We cling to information about ourselves that's superficial and easily accessed because it doesn't tax our self-analytical abilities. What you see is what you get. Anyway, who wants to know all the yucky stuff you may discover about yourself if you poke around too much? What if you don't like what you find?

When I was working at a methadone clinic in which therapy was mandatory, I often was asked by clients why I couldn't just take what they said at face value. Why did everything always have a deeper meaning, and wasn't a cigar sometimes just a cigar? I'd answer that this was sometimes true, but sometimes not true, and that I wanted to be sure. Eventually many of my clients learned to value the search for answers to complicated internal questions because of how satisfying these answers were and how much they enlightened and enriched their lives. After all, when you learn something new about yourself, if you don't want to believe it, you don't have to. But what you don't know about yourself *can* hurt you.

Conscious material is **uncomplicated** and **easily understood.**

In our busy lives, we want instant information and easy answers. Let's face it, humans are awfully bull-headed and too often willing to stay that way. Sadly, our culture is not one in which the journey rather than the destination and striving to maximize our emotional potential are highly prized, except in the most superficial ways. Instead, we incline toward right-or-wrong thinking and good-or-bad behavior. Although there is value in making clear distinctions, as a total mindset such polarization is sorely lacking in breadth, depth, and nuance and not very useful in living a quality life.

It's easy to see why people prefer simplistic to complex. Give us too much information and we become confused and overwhelmed. Forget the questions, just give us the right answers. And, keep it simple, will ya!

How much we value complexity or the lack of it is also often a matter of temperament and upbringing. Children are born curious. They like to explore and ask endless questions. If parents support our appropriate inquisitiveness and encourage us to investigate and understand our world, we don't become intimated by tasks being difficult or complex. We keep going because we want to understand, purely for self-satisfaction. Alternately, if our parents scold us for being inquisitive or make it seem as if we're doing something wrong by being curious, we tend to reign it in so as not to get into trouble. As adults, we might lean toward what's easily grasped on the surface because, wrongly, it seems like the "right" thing to do.

Conscious material can screen out **emotional discomfort.**

Emotional discomfort is what most of us filter out of consciousness. Fear of that discomfort makes a powerful gatekeeper. Maybe we can tolerate a bit of unfamiliarity, rooting around in the dark corners of our minds, or spending time analyzing what makes us tick even though we tell ourselves we have more important things to do, but we sure don't want to be made to feel upset or unhappy with ourselves. *Au contraire!* Most folks in our culture are seriously disinclined to learn new stuff about themselves that doesn't fit into their pre-existing, carefully molded self-concept. One of our most human traits is seeking out information that is consonant with what appears to be our truths—a process called confirmation bias—and avoiding information that creates dissonance and subsequent emotional distress.

Of course, we're not all created equal due to genetics, experiences, and temperament. An example of our differences is how freely we can speak our mind around people who take feedback well, while walking on eggshells around folks who'd rather be struck by lightning than hear a contrary word about themselves. Individuals who are more open to learning about their blind spots and unknown areas tend to seek out information that's unfamiliar, challenging, or even upsetting, thereby increasing what is known and conscious. They believe they can handle it and do.

Alternately, people who fear self-knowledge go out of their way to keep it locked out of awareness through processes such as denial, rationalizing, intellectualizing, or minimizing. Some folks go so far as to project their deficiencies onto others, such as when a generally grumpy colleague says to you, "Hey, what's wrong—you always seem to have a chip on your shoulder?"

One of the words I often hear from clients who don't care to dig too deeply into their psyches or personal history is "dwell." It is such an apt word and I totally get where they're coming from. They believe that if they start to dig, they'll fall into the hole they've made for themselves, never be able to climb out, and be stuck living there forever. Even touching upon a subject or a memory can make them fear being trapped in it. If you're someone who doesn't want to "dwell" on uncomfortable thoughts or feelings, you're not alone, but that doesn't mean you're in healthy company.

> ### Food for Thought
>
> Are you partial only to information about yourself that's familiar and won't cause you emotional distress? If so, why is that? Why are you so afraid of learning about yourself and being emotionally uncomfortable? What's the down side of staying only with what's conscious and comfortable?

If I stick my fingers in my ears, will that block out what I don't want to know?

Now, you're ready to learn another basic concept that bears upon what we allow in or bar from awareness. The fact is, we tune in to only some of our desires—which we'll call wishes—and tune out others—many of which are fears. Let me use an example outside the realm of food to explain what I mean. Say you're attending college in Vermont, it's the holidays, and you have this intense yearning to travel home to Oklahoma to be with family. Gung ho, you keep telling yourself how much fun you'll have and are totally in touch with your longings for hearth and home. However, lurking outside your consciousness there exists just a tickle of memory of the last few visits to your folks' house. Truth be told, most of the time you were there you were pretty unhappy and couldn't wait to get back to school.

Another way of thinking about this situation is that you have two sets of wishes—a conscious set that is propelling you to go home and an unconscious set that, if you heed it, are warning you not to go. Still with me? One set of wishes produces positive emotions that feel okay to acknowledge. The other set causes fear and makes you uncertain what to do, so you tune out or ignore it.

This example illustrates how the mind works and how we often have wishes and fears about the same subject. You are very aware—highly conscious—of the positive feelings contained in your pleasure about going home, but are barely aware or unaware—partially or completely unconscious—of your negative feelings.

Psychologists call the wishes you're conscious of *mani-fest* ("apparent to the eye or to the mind") and the wishes or fears you're partially conscious or unconscious of *latent* ("present but not active; hidden; concealed"). Most people would swear on a stack of bibles that manifest wishes are all they have. Because they never scratch below the surface of their superficial thoughts and emotions, they believe that everything they're aware of is all that exists. Other people have a vague notion that they harbor darker thoughts and feelings, but recoil because even an inkling of what lurks in the shadows gives them the willies. Their motto is "out of sight, out of mind," which is a pleasant attitude in the short run but a disastrous motto for guiding your life.

I don't mean to make light of how we avoid fears. The truth is, we all do it to a greater or lesser extent. But there's a huge difference between taking a firm stance about not wanting to know all that's going on inside of you and being a genuine seeker of self-knowledge but shying away from some of what you find. The process of knowing yourself is more art than science and is an ongoing, life-long quest. Even those of us who truly wish to know the good, the bad, *and* the ugly about ourselves, find it difficult to acknowledge all our fears, never mind challenging them.

So, now, let's take a look at what we have—conscious or manifest wishes which generally make us feel good, and unconscious or latent fears which generally make us feel uncomfortable. If we are psychologically adventurous and courageous, we acknowledge that both sets of information exist side by side and take it from there. Using the Oklahoma holiday visit example, we'd use a wide-angle lens and view the entire panorama, including all the reasons we want to head home and all the reasons we don't. We wouldn't put more value on one set of wishes than the other, and would use both our brains and our hearts to make an appropriate, informed decision.

Food for Thought

Do you prefer sticking to what you know rather than what you might be concealing from yourself? Why? What do you do when you get in touch with a fear?

Where should I put my money—on my manifest or latent wishes?

If you're like most folks, you might believe that manifest and latent wishes have equal power. After all, they're both products of authentic desire. Moreover, your take on the subject of the conscious and unconscious is compounded by what our culture tells us, especially in the area of motivation. Every motivational speaker I've ever heard exhorts audiences to avoid negative thinking, focus exclusively on

achieving their goals, and visualize themselves succeeding. You know the drill: Fake it til you make it, stay upbeat,
there's no such thing as failure.

Although positive thinking and a can-do mentality absolutely have a place in our lives, the truth is that allowing
yourself to have only "positive" thoughts can really mess
with your mind. I understand where these motivational
speakers are coming from and the direction in which they're
trying to herd their audiences. They're attempting to unstick
people from rigid patterns and clear the way to happiness,
an effort I whole-heartedly applaud.

Frankly, there are some people who think this way
naturally. They are born with superior mental health genes
(that is, among other things, a balanced complement of
neurotransmitters), raised by parents who model optimism,
proactivity and empowerment, and taught from childhood
to feel worthwhile. They see the glass as half full and always seem to look on the bright side. Of course, folks can be
taught to change their thinking as well. That's why I write
books, teach workshops, and provide therapy and coaching.
However, from my 30-plus years of clinical experience, I'd
have to say that maintaining success with "normal" eating
and self-care will not come through putting on a perpetual
happy face and ignoring mixed feelings and fears.

Just the opposite, in fact. Professionally speaking, I can
tell you that what we don't know about ourselves *can* hurt
us deeply. More than that, what we don't know can muscle
out and override what we do know and hijack our happiness, while all the time its power source—fear—remains hidden from awareness. Remember the Wizard of Oz cowering
behind the curtain, quaking at being discovered? That's how
you live when you disregard or discount your fears!

Your fears exist because they're keeping you from harm. When fears are ignored, minimized, intellectualized, or rationalized away, they need to work extra hard to make themselves known in order to do their job of protecting you. Without fear, how the heck would animals, human or otherwise, survive? We need to have doubts and qualms and reservations in order to stay alive. Some fears are more innate than learned (of the dark, strangers, objects larger than ourselves), while other are picked up through exposure to the world (fear of fat is certainly drilled into us by the media and culture at large). Fears are neither bad nor good in and of themselves and often are highly useful when they transmit pertinent information such as the need to keep your feet planted on the curb when a truck is speeding through a red light or the voice that tells you never to contradict your boss no matter what kind of chummy drinking buddies you two have become.

Two problems arise with fear. The first is when we bury our fears because they make us uncomfortable and we don't want to face them. I've had a number of female clients with unaddressed marital issues that made them so uncomfortable that every time they started eating healthfully and began enjoying a positive relationship with food, they slipped back into mindless munching. By funneling their energies into changing their bodies and their habits, they filled up their mental space to avoid considering the rotten state of their union. The discomfort they felt about food was nothing compared to the qualms they felt about acknowledging the need for change in their relationship.

The second way fears can be problematic is when they were adaptive and life-enhancing back in childhood, but now have become maladaptive and self-destructive. There are no shortage of instances where our fears harm us today, rather than help. If we were ignored, humiliated, or hurt as children when we challenged authority, it made sense to keep silent, whereas it makes no sense today to suffer in silence when we are ignored or humiliated by our boss. You can see how early fears were adaptive and helped you survive, so it's not the fears *per se* that are wrong. It's the fact that you still have them when you no longer need them. They were appropriate—essential for survival—in childhood, but are no longer functional in adulthood.

That's why it's so important to be conscious of our fears. We have to know which ones to toss into the trash bin, which ones to treasure because they protect us, and which ones to set aside for the maybe pile. However, and it's a biggie, we can't do this if we believe it's wrong to have fears and, instead, whistle our way through the darkness to avoid the discomfort of thinking about them.

> ### *Food for Thought*
> What are your most prevalent fears? Do you ignore them? Let them run your life? Do you still need them today or are they obsolete?

If I acknowledge my fears, won't that give them too much power?

First off, remember that our fears exist, even if we're not aware of them. Like barricades on a dark road, we may not see them, but we sure know when we crash into them. Contrary to the popular myth that fears are nothing more than errant thoughts, they are often more powerful than our desires, whether we like it or not.

And that's where emotional conflict enters the picture. Recall that most of our wishes and desires are *manifest* and known to us, and too many of our fears are *latent* and outside of awareness. How might that cause internal conflict? It predisposes us to act in one way in response to one set of wishes that are known to us *and* act in the opposite way in response to another set of wishes which are not known to us. Simply put, we suffer from conflict when we say we want one thing and do the opposite over and over again. There's a struggle going on when we put off making decisions or can't break out of rigid, destructive behavior in spite of negative consequences. We're in the thick of internal conflict when we have every reason to attain realistic goals yet fail repeatedly to do so.

The psychological description of an unconscious conflict is *when your intentions don't align with your behavior.* If you say you want to be healthy and eat mostly unhealthy foods, there's a conflict brewing. If you say you love yourself and rarely get enough sleep and allow your stress level to go through the roof, you've got a conflict going on. You're not stupid, lazy, or unmotivated. Isn't it a relief to know that? You're merely conflicted!

The result of intentions clashing with behavior is not reaching your goals or, alternately, attaining them briefly, then letting success slip away. If this happens frequently, look for mixed or contradictory feelings yanking the strings behind the curtain. When feelings are conflicted—wish versus fear—we're pulled in opposite directions. Either the tugs are equal and we do nothing (insist we want a job, but fail to network, send out applications, or read the classifieds) or we do one thing, then undo it (snag a job, but self-sabotage and lose it).

Procrastination is a perfect example of internal, unconscious conflict and one with which many disregulated eaters are all too familiar. I love to explain to clients that they're not sloths for not doing what they intend to do, especially what's on their endless to-do lists. Here they've thought for most, if not all, of their lives that they were defective or incompetent when they didn't get things done. The truth is, they're only ambivalent!

Most of us blame ourselves for being lazy, but, frankly, I've yet to meet a truly lazy person in my clinical practice. What I have met by the hundreds are folks who have unconscious, contradictory feelings. You know the dilemmas. You tell yourself you should exercise, but never step on the treadmill that's still in the unopened box in the garage. You want to clean the house, but exhausted Super Woman that you are, end up watching *Seinfeld* reruns and feeling guilty. Some people almost make a career out of procrastination, then beat themselves up unmercifully for failing to get things done or achieve their goals. If you're one of these people, take heart. Procrastination is nothing more than conflicted feelings that get played out in opposing directions. Once conflicts are identified and understood, they'll begin to resolve themselves, and you'll start managing life more consciously and effectively rather than giving power to what's been unconsciously driving you.

What we call self-sabotage and relapse are also by-products of unconscious, opposing feelings. You barrel along toward success and reach it, but when your hidden fears kick in, your choo choo goes hurtling backwards. This one-step-forward-two-steps-back pattern takes its toll. More often than not, after playing out this struggle more than a few times, you give up. The key to sustained success is understanding that self-sabotage involves two sets of motivations both vying for time. First you succeed, which meets one set of desires, then you stop yourself from succeeding, which meets another set of desires or fears. In psych parlance, this is called an *approach-avoidance syndrome*. Only by recognizing that you're caught between competing wishes and fears, can you finally stop zig-zagging and head in one direction toward lasting success.

In trying to improve their relationship with food, many disregulated eaters follow their appetite cues for a while and glory in how their bodies feel. Then something happens which causes them distress—they have a disagreement with a neighbor, lose a big work account, or receive the cold shoulder from a friend—and suddenly all they want to do is eat sugar and fat to feel better. That is, they *want* to eat junk food to reduce distress and *don't want* to because they have been feeling the best they've felt in years. That's one kind of conflict, and the tension between the two opposing wishes—to feel good with food and to feel good without it—causes them to fear they'll snap in two.

Another kind of conflict occurs when a person goes to the gym for a while and starts to see her body grow gradually fitter. Soon people begin to notice and comment on how well she looks, and she finds herself feeling oddly uncomfortable. She kind of likes the praise and kind of doesn't. Eventually she tells herself she has no time for the gym, but the real reason she drops out is because she has underlying discomfort about the attention she's receiving.

The way out of these clashes is to acknowledge both feelings and work on coming to a conscious resolution. Too many disregulated eaters know they're conflicted but shy away from working through their dilemmas. They end up acting out in ways that are anything but in their best interest. I can't say what the "right" resolution would be in any of the above situations, but I can tell you that being aware of both sets of feelings and experiencing and dealing with them will put whatever the issue is to rest.

Must I spend the rest of my life in analysis to resolve my internal conflicts?

Although therapy can fairly quickly help you identify the pushes and pulls within you, you can learn to recognize them yourself with time, practice, and patience. To begin with, you may believe you shouldn't have mixed feelings or ever feel conflicted. It's natural to want emotions to line up so you can handle them one at a time because life is simpler that way.

Plus, looking around, you may assume that everyone else is certain about what they want and what they're doing (ha!) and believe that life should be as easy as it appears to be for them. You may think you're the only one floundering, the only one who keeps having the same struggles and doubts over and over. The truth is that people who are successful and fulfilled generally aren't devoid of internal conflict—that's not possible because we all have ambivalences to a greater or lesser extent. Instead, wise folk identify their hidden fears and resolve their conflicts so they can move forward and stay there. Moreover, if you surround yourself with people who have a right-wrong mindset and, of course, always think they're right, you may feel like the odd person out with your doubts and ambivalence. The truth is, you may be far more mentally healthy than more rigid-thinking folks (even if they're your parents!). Remember, a person who acts as if they're never wrong is a person driven by fear and shame.

Another problem with mixed feelings is that they can just plain feel yucky. They fill us with doubt, uncertainty, and insecurity. We want so desperately to *be* right and *do* right that we yearn for "the way," "the secret," and "the answer." We forgo resolving internal conflict because the process is too messy and unsettling. Better to close down our brains and have someone else tell us what to do!

Sometimes we're ashamed that we have contradictory feelings about things such as loving our parents or children, taking care of ourselves, or seeking financial success. When we're ashamed, we avoid looking squarely at what we feel and pretend we don't feel it. Other times we're thrown into such a tizzy by conflicting feelings that we're sure our heads will explode. The only response that comes out loud and clear is the urge to shut off the conflict and act as if it doesn't exist. Often followed by the urge to binge!

But, conflict remains within us. It's like leaving on the TV with the sound muted. The program is still going, even if you can't hear it. So, you might as well face the music—life is full of internal tugs of war, so get used to them and learn how to benefit from the valuable information they bring so you can better manage them.

Food for Thought

What are your current conflicts about food, weight or self-care? How have you tried to resolve them? What happens when they're unresolved? What better ideas do you now have for resolving them?

I want to skip to what to do about my conflicts, but I'm afraid I'll miss something important.

That's the ticket. Now you're getting the idea: You're recognizing your mixed feelings. But, not to fret. You're almost ready to be introduced to the seven keys that will unlock the dilemmas that are preventing you from eating "normally," exercising regularly, and taking exemplary care of yourself. The only additional construct needed is understanding what a *core conflict* is.

First, let me tell you what it's not. It isn't a *minor everyday* occurrence, such as trying to decide if you should answer your emails now or after lunch—not the mundane, relatively inconsequential, easily resolved, and quickly forgotten uncertainties that fill your day. You know you're talking minor conflict when neither side of the divide generates much emotional heat.

Another kind of internal struggle that is not a core conflict is in the realm of the *irresolvable*. Questions about the meaning of life and the existence of God fall into this category. You may never come to a conclusion because these are philosophical, existential questions. The Big Mysteries of Life. After all, who ever said we were supposed to have all the answers? For the most part, we learn to live with wavering opinions on these subjects and with similar ambiguities and uncertainties. They make us feel tolerably uncomfortable, and only occasionally create severe emotional disturbance.

Core conflicts, on the other hand, are the rock bottom reasons (other than biological) that we do or don't do things, the unresolved dilemmas that mire us in unhealthy attitudes and destructive behavioral patterns. They speak to our identity, worth and value, the essence of who we are, how we view and fit into the world, and the way we wish to live our lives. However, once core conflicts are resolved, intent and behavior align more naturally and completely. Some people wait until they're nearing the end of life to figure out what it was all about. Why wait? By nailing down the answers to several key questions right now, you'll have a better chance to enjoy the life ahead of you.

HOMEWORK

Write out these answers for yourself.

1. What did you learn in this chapter about the conflicts that may prevent you from sustaining positive eating, fitness, and self-care behaviors?

2. What ideas or concepts were new to you?

3. Which new concepts or ideas made you feel better or more hopeful?

4. Which new concepts or ideas made you feel uncomfortable or anxious?

5. What specific actions can you take to resolve your conflicts?

---

[1] Beck, A., Bennett, P. & Wall, P. (2002) *Communication Studies: The Essential Introduction,* New York:Routledge, p. 172-3

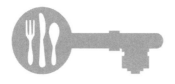

THE SEVEN KEYS TO A PERMANENT, POSITIVE RELATIONSHIP WITH FOOD

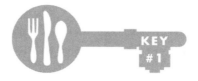

CHAPTER 4

CREATE LASTING CHANGE

(Can't I Just Wish Upon a Star?)

We all want change to happen—like yesterday. Believe me, I wish I could wave a magic wand and heal you all instantly. Having had food problems and body issues galore during the first half of my life, I know how low they can bring you, how darkly they can color your entire existence. If I could turn around your eating lickety split through my words, I'd do it in a New York minute. But I can't. No one can.

Research has made amazing discoveries about genetics, hormones, and the biochemistry of eating. These scientific strides are teaching us that there's no one-size-fits-all cause of eating problems, and that weight gain and loss are far more complex than we ever dreamed. We're also learning about the cues in our environment that trigger unwanted eating and how to change and respond to those cues differently.

Psychotherapy and psycho-education also play a major role in improving motivation and resolving the myriad issues related to food abuse. For now, all we can do is learn as much as possible about food and eating and accept that going from disregulated to "normal" eating is going to take a long time—although there are actions we can take to speed up or slow down the process.

When it comes to change, we're all wearing cute, little baby shoes and taking awkward baby steps. So, are you ready to tie up your laces and get to work? Good. For starters, how about creating a psychological shift right this minute. Ready? Okay, instruct yourself never again to think or ask someone, even an expert, "How long will this process take?" Instead, spend a minute reassuring yourself that if you take enough baby steps (remember, there's nothing but!) in the direction of "normal" eating—and don't give up—you'll eventually get there. This shift takes the focus off your distant goal and puts it where it belongs and will do you more good: on the process of change itself. The same is true of becoming more physically fit and taking better care of yourself. You don't need to know *when* you'll get there, but you do need to know *how*. Simply accept that if you keep moving forward, change will happen gradually in its own sweet time.

Let's start by exploring your unconscious mixed feelings about change. Your brain is saying, *I want to be a "normal" eater more than I've ever wanted anything in my life. And I want it as soon as possible. That's it, case closed.* Well, not really—case still open! What we believe about the process of healing makes all the difference in whether or not we'll heal. Again, note that I'm talking not about the *what* of change but the *how*.

At the root of any endeavor is not only a desire to reach a goal, but expectations about the how and when of success. It's this *process of how change occurs* that disregulated eaters tend to have a slew of beliefs and feelings about that are at odds with each other.

Food for Thought

Consider how you or people you know have made significant, lasting attitudinal or behavioral change. What are the key elements of the process? What are your beliefs about change? What's your evidence for these beliefs?

Why can't change happen in a jiffy?

If expecting change to happen overnight underlies your approach to navigating through life, you're going to be bummed out every time change takes its own pokey time, which it is sure to do. I understand where you're coming from: we live in a culture that puts undue emphasis on the end result rather than the means to get there. The concepts of hard work, patience, and incremental change seem old-fashioned these days. Instead, we're bombarded with seductive stories about overnight success. Even health insurance companies have gotten into the act by insisting on shorter and shorter recovery times. Better yet, take some pills to speed up the process and you're good to go.

Wishing that change would happen quickly is understandable. The only question is: Does your experience support that behavioral change happens quickly? If so, I want some of what you're smoking, because *my* reality says that change nearly always happens in fits and starts and never quickly enough.

The name for the misguided wish that permanent change will happen without ongoing effort is *magical thinking*. Technically, magical thinking is a psychology term describing the way we ascribe cause and effect when there is none, especially in childhood. All of us engaged in magical thinking as youngsters, because we understood so little of how the world actually worked. For example, magical thinking is at work when a child mistakenly believes she's the cause of her parents not getting along or when a pre-teen thinks that if he only behaves like a good boy, Mom won't yell at him so much when she's drinking. There's nothing remotely wrong with this kind of primitive belief for kids; it's normal for a child whose brain is only partially developed and whose life experience is severely limited. There is everything wrong with continuing to hold on to magical thinking about change as an adult with a fully developed brain and decades of experience.

Luckily we're able to shift our beliefs, including our cognitions about change. Doing so will open your eyes to an enlightened way of thinking about transformation that actually may speed it along. In fact, just viewing the change process more realistically will increase your confidence, self-compassion, and the likelihood of moving forward and progressing. Thinking more realistically will open the doors to more rational action, that is, those that are evidence-based and in your long-term best interest. Can you see the paradox at work here? Hoping for a quick fix slows down your healing, while acknowledging that change usually happens at a crawl, hastens it!

Food for Thought

Do you engage in magical thinking? Has it helped or hurt in reaching your eating, weight, and self-care goals? Are you ready to give it up and become more realistic? If not, what's holding you back?

How come my brain didn't grow up with the rest of me?

Let me start by offering complete assurance that most of your brain is probably working just fine, but your understanding about change may need a bit of an adjustment. Transforming beliefs is like updating yourself regarding new technology. You're not walking around carrying a sundial, are you? To enhance your life, it's time to ditch magical thinking, get with the program, and get in synch with reality.

Exactly how we come to retain immature, irrational beliefs as an adult is worth examining. Most of what we think, we learn from our families, particularly from our parents. Here are 10 questions about how parents view and model behavioral change to illuminate the origin of your views today. Did your parents:

1. Express impatience and frustration when learning or teaching new things?

2. Start to change, give up, and try again with the same failed strategies?

3. Despair or become enraged when change failed to happen quickly or quickly enough?

4. Model setting realistic goals, valuing incremental change, and taking baby steps?

5. Ask for help and support when they needed it or insist on going it alone?

6. Avoid changing by coerce or manipulate others into changing so that they didn't have to?

7. Use shaming or punishment to motivate you, themselves, or each other to change?

8. Consider success nothing less than perfection or think in terms of success/failure, winning/losing, or all/nothing?

9. Follow a pattern of achieving a goal only to revert to old behaviors?

10. Help you reach goals in a reasonable, fair, comfortable way that felt good to you?

Parenting is a tough job and most Moms and Dads either follow how their parents raised them or react by doing the opposite. Neither approach is constructive. Effective parenting comes from self-knowledge, adaptability, openness to learning new skills, ongoing reflection, and focusing on what is in the best interest of the child. The fact is, if parents are unskilled at creating and sustaining change (maybe no one ever taught *them* how), it's highly unlikely that they will be effective teachers. So, not only does a child not learn appropriate ways to think about and engage in change, but she ends up learning unproductive ways that continue to plague her right into adulthood.

This issue of role modeling reminds me of how I learned to ski, trailing behind a friend who was maybe one skill level ahead of me. Years later, when I got around to taking formal lessons, the instructor shook his head sadly as he checked out my form on the slopes. He then proceeded to help me unlearn all the incorrect habits from my friend and teach me the basics from scratch. I felt silly going the beginners' route after a decade on the slopes, but his method worked. I became a decent skier by shedding the wrong techniques and learning the right ones.

This is the model you may have to follow if you want your head on straight regarding change. You can improve at anything—including eating and caring for your body—with patience and practice. The place to start is by letting go of unrealistic, unhealthy attitudes about change and replacing them with realistic, healthy ones.

Food for Thought

What helpful attitudes about behavioral change did you learn from family members? What unhelpful attitudes? Which irrational beliefs about change might be most difficult to let go of? What rational beliefs will replace them?

Where exactly do I go wrong in thinking about how behavioral change happens?

Although intellectually we may realize that anything worth doing takes a long time and lots of elbow grease, the still immature aspect of self may blind its eyes to a truth which makes us feel inadequate, inept, and convinced that reaching our goals is just too darned hard.

To illustrate how thinking about behavioral change can go awry, let's take a look at some of the basic behaviors you may need to engage in to become a "normal" eater:

• Eating only when hungry and stopping when satisfied

- Planning meals or snacks ahead rather than grabbing food on the go
- Taking small portions and eating slowly
- Thinking in terms of "more or less nutritious" rather than "good or bad" foods
- Eating throughout the day, rather than starving until dinner and bingeing at night
- Spending time shopping for and preparing healthy meals
- Avoiding a diet based on sugars, fats and heavily salted or processed foods
- Drinking water for the most part, not soda or heavily sweetened juice
- Managing stress and distress effectively
- Eating mindfully without doing other tasks
- Focusing on eating, not weight
- Eating with goals of enjoyment and satisfaction
- Getting enough sleep so that hunger and satiation hormones are in balance

These are just some of the basic practices that over time will lead to achieving a positive relationship with food. Depending upon the severity of disregulated eating, these basics may take many months to a few years to become habitual. Be wary of trying to do all these practices at once and hoping for too much too soon. Because of an all-or-nothing mindset, you might feel overwhelmed by what you believe you *must* do to become a flawless eater which is sure to generate mixed feelings: While part of you is hankering to step on the gas pedal, another part will be slamming on the brakes so you can stay exactly where you are.

The problem is not merely one of being conflicted, but of being aware of only the manifest or positive reasons you wish to change, and being totally out of touch with the latent or uncomfortable reasons you wish not to. Positive motivation—desiring to eat better and become healthier encourages us and gives us hope. On the other hand, doubts about putting a plan into action and actually getting going can make us feel so overwhelmed that we tend to brush them aside. This all adds up to wondering why we should bother trying to succeed to begin with. Sound familiar?

Changing Erroneous Beliefs

I've been talking in generalizations here, so let's get down to specific *belief errors* about the change process which might be holding you back.

BELIEF ERROR: I'll change all my "bad" behaviors at once and be free of them.

Many disregulated eaters bite off more than they can chew, literally and figuratively. Instead of saying they'll try to change one or two behaviors at a time, they want to eradicate all their errant ways in one fell swoop—stop smoking and start exercising, cut out drinking and begin meditation, avoid eating meat and go totally organic. I'm exhausted setting down these goals. Can you imagine trying to do them all at once?

This kind of all-or-nothing thinking reminds me of a friend I knew decades ago who tried to get healthy all at once. First, she stopped drinking, and after several weeks managed to get in the swing of ordering club soda or coffee rather than booze. Then she gave up cigarettes because she mostly smoked when she drank. Finally, when she was nicotine *and* alcohol free for a month or so, she tackled her eating by cutting out sweets and cutting back on portion size. However, by then she was a jittery, ornery mess. After another week or so on the straight and (very) narrow, she succumbed to sneaking a cigarette from a colleague, and all hell broke loose. Within a week, she'd gone back to smoking, drinking, and abusing food. The moral of the story? Don't try to tackle more than is reasonable at one time. The fact is, we're programmed to change behaviors slowly.

Better beliefs:

- I can manage changing one habit at a time.
- A great start in getting healthy is eliminating just one unhealthy habit.
- I have the patience and motivation to tackle one issue, then another.

BELIEF ERROR: I can change my habits quickly and easily.

Many people pooh-pooh the idea of taking baby steps and underestimate the time it takes to alter long-standing behavioral patterns. In the case of changing habits, success is more likely to be ours if we think about longer rather than shorter time periods (as well as harder rather than easier work). Plan on a lengthy but realistic timeline, then be surprised if progress moves at a faster clip than expected. Your best bet is to take off the pressure and remind yourself that you'll get there when you get there.

Better beliefs:

- Habits take time to change and that's okay.

- I don't mind doing whatever hard work is necessary for success.

- If I put in effort on a consistent basis, in time I can change any behavior I want to.

BELIEF ERROR: Based on my past, I probably won't succeed at reaching my health goals or, even if I do, I won't be able to sustain them.

Disregulated eaters spend an inordinate amount of mental time looking backward and forward, and very little in the present, the only place where you can actually *make* change. If you've spent years or decades battling weight or yo-yoing between restricting and overeating, it's no surprise that you look at your history and mistake it for your future. Rather than be disappointed (or disappoint others) again, your fears and hopelessness warn you not to even bother trying, so you don't.

But, alter the story, and you'll change the ending. Spending years dieting and regaining weight is nothing like learning and practicing the rules of "normal" eating. The only thing that dieting and intuitive eating have in common is that they both involve food.

Better beliefs:

- I can learn to eat "normally" because it's nothing like dieting.

- I can learn to be comfortable with food and my body.

- I have new thinking and new skills that will sustain my new health habits.

BELIEF ERROR: It's too hard to exercise regularly, eat healthfully, and do all the things I need to do for ongoing self-care.

Many disregulated eaters have feelings about hard work which arc wildly from one extreme to the other. On the one hand, they glory in accomplishing tasks and are happy when they've done them flawlessly. On the other, they're easily overwhelmed by what they believe they "need" to do and procrastinate like the dickens. Because many consider lack of productivity shameful, they can't let go of the Puritan work ethic, though they don't seem able to live by it either. They believe they *should* like hard work and work hard, but deep in their hearts wish they didn't have to.

The error in this belief is that eating well, exercising regularly, and consistent self-care seem like work. Ask people who do it automatically and most will shrug and insist that they enjoy taking good care of their bodies. The idea that it's hard work might not have occurred to them because they're concentrating on the benefits they're receiving, not the effort they're expending. Other folks who take good care of themselves will agree that it involves focus and energy, but they'll also smile and tell you that it's so worthwhile, the effort hardly matters.

It can be difficult getting started eating well and exercising, but once you do these things more regularly, they simply become part of life and you miss them when you don't do them. After a while, your body feels great and you associate positive self-care with positive feelings, not with hard work.

Better beliefs:

• I can decide how I want to view putting effort into the goals I want to reach.

• Eating better and getting fit can be enjoyable and bring enormous pleasure.

• Activities which are initially hard become easier over time.

BELIEF ERROR: I'm just not good at taking care of myself.

Aside from knowing how to set realistic goals and pace yourself, in order to succeed you need two essential life skills. The first is *frustration tolerance* which means putting up with—and ignoring or overriding—the discomfort you feel when the going gets rough. The second is the *ability to delay gratification*, which means being okay with not receiving a reward right away and, instead, recognizing that by pressing forward, it will come. Delaying gratification means not expecting to feel so great as you labor, but knowing that you will find your pot of gold at the end of the rainbow.

Sure, the fortunate among us learned frustration tolerance and how to delay gratification as children, but that doesn't mean these skills aren't learnable at any age. By forcing yourself to tolerate frustration and delay gratification—encouraging yourself to go to the gym though it's raining because you *know* how great you'll feel afterwards, spending time making a healthy meal because you *know* how satisfied you'll feel, and the like—you'll be so tickled with having the ability to take care of yourself that you'll want to act in your best interest again and again.

Better beliefs:

- If other people can learn to take better care of themselves, I can too.

- I can learn how to defer gratification and tolerate frustration.

- There is no reason on earth why I can't take excellent care of myself.

BELIEF ERROR: *I have to eat, exercise, and take care of myself perfectly or why bother.*

I hope you're smartening up enough to see the fallacy in this belief. Why would anyone need to be flawless? What a crazy idea that imperfect beings should or could behave perfectly—believing that you can never have a sweet or miss a day of exercise. The thought of only "being good" and doing it for life is enough to make any sane person want to shoot hot fudge into their veins til they're unconscious, so ease up.

By deciding when enough is enough, eating well, exercising regularly, and maintaining self-care will fall nicely into place. If you miss one night of taking your vitamins, so what? Resume the next day. Can't do your usual gym workout, so do a mini-version. I'll take "enough" over perfection any day. I know I can achieve "enough" and can't ever get to perfection, so I don't even try to reach such a silly goal.

Better beliefs:

- I will do just what is enough for me.

- I won't waste time being rigid and going for unattainable perfection.

- By doing what is enough for me in the realm of food, activity, and self-care—and no more!—I'll be able to sustain these positive behaviors.

BELIEF ERROR: I can't stop until I reach my goals.

Who says? Too often we set a goal, then keep pushing toward it even though we've arrived at a nice stopping point along the way. For example, you may decide you *have* to become a vegan, when it will bring you far more pleasure being a vegetarian. People who are driven to never stop until they achieve a goal—even if it doesn't feel good or causes them harm—are generally operating with an all-or-nothing mindset that makes them unhappy at either end of the spectrum. At the outset, you're missing the present because you're focused on future success, and when you get there, you're terrified of holding onto what you've achieved.

A better way to make decisions about goals is to set the bar low, and when you get to a reasonable stopping point, rest and see how it feels. I was at a gym in a hotel and a mere slip of a girl limped in and over to an all-in-one weight machine. It was painful to watch as she pushed herself through each set of leg exercises. She could barely stand on her bad leg, never mind lift weights with it. I wanted to drag her away from the gym and sit her down and tell her that what her body needed was not a beating but rest, and that she would be much better off if she'd put her foot up for a while until whatever was wrong with it had healed. I bet she had a goal to go to the gym every day and wasn't going to let anything get in her way, not even a bum leg. That's what being too enamored with goals can do to you.

Better beliefs:

- I can set goals, try to achieve them, then stop any time I want.

- I will only pursue goals I want, not those I feel I should pursue.

- Meeting a goal isn't nearly as important as taking care of myself and listening to my care-taking voice.

BELIEF ERROR: *I won't be satisfied even if I reach my goals, so why should I bother trying?*

Being goal-oriented is a terrific trait and works for *some* people, but you've heard of having too much of a good thing, haven't you? Some people are *never* truly satisfied with themselves or what they achieve. They set a realistic goal, accomplish it, but still are bothered by not feeling the sense of satisfaction they hoped to feel. Or they experience it only fleetingly, then feel let down. Instead of trying to figure out why they so need the headiness of success, they set another goal, then another and another.

This more-is-better mentality is often what leads to overeating—if one donut tastes delish, then three will be a delish trifecta. If everyone's oohing and ahing over your 30-pound weight loss, how awesome would it be to lose 10 or 20 more?

Disregulated eaters who tend to be obsessive with goals may do better not setting any. They may make more rapid progress by taking a day at a time and focussing on small satisfactions: How good it feels to walk rather than drive to a friend's house, how lovely it is to eat some tangy cut up fruit rather than drift hungrily through the afternoon ravenous for dinner, or to take a yoga class rather than your bike club's six-hour ride.

Some people are satisfied with everyday accomplishments, while others remain unsatisfied no matter how much they do. Start paying attention to what satisfies you. Think small and your smiles will be bigger.

Better beliefs:

- I can feel satisfied and that I've gone far enough at any point in trying to reach my goals.

- I will focus on getting pleasure from small satisfactions rather than looking for big ones.

- When I've achieved my goals, I will relax and enjoy having achieved them.

BELIEF ERROR: Being accountable for myself is a drag.

On some level, we'd all rather blame other people for our shortcomings than hold ourselves accountable. I know there are times that I would! It's hard to stay on top of being responsible for your actions 24/7 and it's a release and relief to occasionally place the blame outside of one's self.

In general, disregulated eaters have a mixed relationship with accountability. A typical client—of any age—thinks she should have been able to change by now and laments the fact that she's still wrestling with food and psychological demons. However, she also makes excuses for why she's not changing. She may blame genes, stress, or relationships. What a contradiction, huh? My job is to not buy into clients' justifications, but to gently remind them that if they can't manage their lives well enough to eat mindfully once a day, they're not likely to become a "normal" eater.

Accountability means honest assessment without judgment. By feeling proud of our self-care efforts—no matter how small—we no longer seek to place blame for not engaging in them.

Better beliefs:

- I am the architect of my life and that thrills me.

- I can be accountable yet non-judgmental and compassionate toward myself.

- Being accountable for myself is a pleasure and makes me proud.

BELIEF ERROR: I want to change without being uncomfortable.

The fear of being emotionally or physically uncomfortable is one of the biggest reasons disregulated eaters are conflicted about change. Somewhere along the way you've mistakenly learned that you can get something for nothing. Do you still dream of that magic solution that will transform you overnight? Oh, it's a grand dream, but it's pie in the sky.

Rather than think of discomfort as negative, try thinking of it as the pre-eminent precursor to change. Along with awareness, discomfort is the major ingredient of going from being this way to becoming that way. It's the key to shifting from being the same to being different. It's simply part of the journey.

Better beliefs:

- I can tolerate being uncomfortable to achieve worthwhile goals.

- Stretching myself can be mildly uncomfortable, but it won't kill me.

• I can decide when to tone down or amp up discomfort as needed.

Food for Thought

What are 3-5 new, positive beliefs about change that will help you move forward?

I wouldn't be at all surprised if you were a bit stunned at how complicated creating lasting transformation really is. You may not even have realized how your conflicts have kept you ambivalent about change. Perhaps some ideas I've presented are triggering discomfort or confusion. That's okay. Take a few deep breaths and relax. Remember, discomfort is a pre-requisite to change, and confusion opens the door to new ways of understanding. We're talking evolution here, not revolution! So let yourself evolve.

I hope this chapter gives you a deeper appreciation of how revamping beliefs about change will help you achieve better health without backsliding.

Meet Katie and Her Conflict

The facts:

When Katie first entered my office, with her hair casually pulled back into a bouncing ponytail, gazing at me with doe eyes and childlike hopefulness, I thought she was much younger than her stated age of 26. After introducing herself, she giggled and told me that she was ready for me to "fix" her eating problems. Katie explained that she lived at home with her surgeon mother and bank VP father because she was between jobs. She'd been trained as a teacher but never had worked as one. She said her parents were going all out with their contacts to help find the right position for her, stressing that she "really, really wanted something that would be a good fit."

She described her eating problem as trying to eat healthily like her parents, but failing constantly by sneaking food into her room or going out with friends and binge-eating. Right now, she said she was the skinniest she'd ever been, but she feared she could easily shoot up 30 pounds if she wasn't "super careful." She confessed that she occasionally purged after overeating. She acknowledged that her parents were paying for therapy and that they had pressured her into several previous diet programs when her weight had ballooned up.

Katie added that her parents said they were unhappy that she was living at home, but did everything for her, including her laundry and meal preparation. Making sure that she was well taken care of was how they showed their love. At one point in the first session she half-joked that it was too bad they couldn't fix her eating problems the way they fixed everything else.

Katie's conflict:

Katie's parents did so much for her that she was clueless about how to get where she wanted to go on her own. Her conflict was that she wanted to change, but expected it to simply happen without ongoing effort. Although I never doubted Katie's sincere desire to eat "normally," I recognized that she had little tolerance for frustration, held an immature expectation of other people swooping in to take care of her, and was looking to me (as she did to her parents) as a savior. In short, she wanted the gain without the pain.

The resolution:

My work with Katie went slowly, in fits and starts. In the beginning we talked a lot about what made her overeat, and I repeatedly normalized how trying to be good all the time triggers bingeing for many people. Most of the time, Katie had difficulty answering my questions, exhibiting little patience with self-reflection. She was frustrated that I wouldn't give her answers to questions, missing the point that looking for our own answers is what we all have to do as mature adults. Katie was torn, stuck in a transitional stage that usually happens in adolescence, when we stop looking to others for help and start taking pride in thinking and doing for ourselves. Because her parents continually over-indulged her, she had never successfully negotiated this stage of development. She had no idea that she could find herself a job and recover from her eating problems if she would simply become more accountable.

Several months into the therapy, Katie was still waiting for me to cure her and even kidded that if I were *really* a smart therapist, I would have fixed her binge eating by now. With much encouragement, she finally found a job as a teacher, but complained bitterly about having to get up early, take work home, and discipline unruly children. I was her best cheerleader and let her "borrow" my belief in her until she had more of it herself. We talked a great deal about her growing pride in managing to drag herself to school every day and how pleasurable feelings about her accomplishments could offset the negatives of the job. I was teaching her to tolerate frustration, delay gratification, and look to pride as an incentive.

Months later, I knew change was afoot when Katie told her parents she was saving money to get her own apartment. She still wasn't crazy about the hardships of her job, but she was now looking at them more as challenges, felt determined to stick things out, and expressed a quiet pleasure in taking care of herself. She had stopped all purging and binged less frequently.

Katie wasn't necessarily enjoying the hard work and discomfort of resisting food cravings, but she finally recognized that nothing she wanted was going to happen unless she gave up her rescue fantasy. Over the course of our work, she became less conflicted about how change happens and more clear that she could ask for help when she really needed it, but that making progress was basically up to her.

HOMEWORK

Write out these answers for yourself.

1. What is the most important thing you learned in this chapter about how change happens?

2. What ideas and concepts about change were new to you?

3. Which new concepts or ideas made you feel better or more hopeful?

4. Which new concepts or ideas made you feel uncomfortable or anxious?

5. Based on this chapter, what specific actions will you take to be more realistic about the change process?

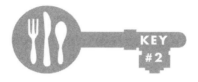

CHAPTER 5

MAKE CONSCIOUS CHOICES

(How Come When I Lash Out, I Hit Me?)

Many disregulated eaters—often unconsciously—dislike anyone telling them what to do. This is true even when that anyone is little old you! For example, you tell yourself you *should* eat a healthy meal but instead scarf down junk food. Or that you *have to* go to the gym, but instead tell your workout buddy you're too tired, and end up surfing the internet and watching mindless TV. Sometimes you have a vague sense of your healthful intention as you're doing its antithesis; others times, feelings of shame and guilt wash over you for not following through on what you believe you *should* have done and—once again—didn't do.

Then, because you don't understand the dynamics that are taking place in your psyche, you likely give yourself a stern reprimand for being lazy or unmotivated, continually asking yourself, "What's wrong with me? Why can't I make good on my intentions?" This disappointment leads to making new promises to change behaviors that you know you're seriously unlikely to keep.

Over years or even decades, this pattern can grind you down. I know because I engaged in it myself during the first half of my life. It feels as if there are two warring factions living within you engaging in continuous battle. You don't want to give up your positive intentions for taking better care of yourself, but you also can't seem to stop sabotaging your eating and self-care goals. My heart goes out to you. Really it does. So read on to discover the key to resolving this dilemma and know that with a bit of understanding and determination you can extricate yourself from it. The good news is that by resolving conflicted feelings about making wise choices regarding food, fitness, and self-care, you'll become more capable of reaching and sustaining your goals.

Food for Thought

Do you follow a pattern of sometimes engaging in positive behaviors, then suddenly or gradually stopping them? How long has this been going on? Are you puzzled by your see-saw actions and attribute them to laziness or defectiveness? What actions have you taken to stop this swinging pendulum? Are you open to new thinking about changing this pattern once and for all?

How can I want so much to be good to myself and still treat myself so horridly?

How indeed? There really is a simple explanation for this seemingly bizarre process, so bear with me while I throw out some ideas that may be new (and even surprising) to you. In part, the culprits responsible for your yo-yoing patterns are common, seemingly innocuous words like should, must, need to, have to and am supposed to—words you repeat to yourself about a gazillion times a day. I've never spoken with a disregulated eater without these words peppering our discussion. I wouldn't be surprised if they order themselves around in their dreams!

I have one client who is forever putting on her most earnest face and prodding herself to *do* something—pay her tax bill, mulch her garden, listen to a yoga CD—but she never does. Well, actually, she does engage in some of these tasks occasionally, even completing the most dire of them, but only at the very last minute because she's terrified of what would happen if she didn't do them. However, the ones like mulching the garden or relaxing to a yoga CD, she rarely gets around to doing.

I learned an important lesson about words like *should* and *must*—called *external motivators*—while working at the methadone clinic in Boston decades ago. A novice therapist, I was pushing a client, a heroin addict, to join one of the clinic's groups. I insisted, "Mike, you really need some support." No sooner had he heard the word "need" than his face got beet red and he shook his finger in my face and hissed, "Don't you ever, *ever* tell me what I need to do!" Although I apologized for my *faux pas*, I can tell you that this one word ended our discussion—and he never allowed me to bring up joining the group again.

What triggered Mike was what triggers you when you badger yourself with what you "should" or "need" to do. No one wants to be pressured to do what someone else wants them to do. Telling someone they *must, ought to, etc.* is demeaning and disrespectful and it's natural for us to have a defensive reaction to these authoritarian words. Even if we recognize that people have our best interests at heart (as I did with my clinic client), when they're telling us what we *must* do, we can't help but bristle.

You're no exception and neither am I. Stop and think about your reaction when a boss, teacher, or parent speaks to you as if you're under their command and uses words that give you the message that you have no say in a matter. You may be so used to certain people speaking to you (and everyone else) this way that you don't even realize how inappropriate it is. So, take a minute and see if you can identify the feelings these words trigger in you.

Food for Thought

How often do you use the words *should, must, have to, need to, supposed to,* and *ought to*? Do you insist that you *shouldn't* eat certain foods, then eat them anyway? How do you feel when you speak to yourself this way? Why do you choose these words over more appropriate ways of expressing intention?

Why do we get so bent out of shape when we're told what's "right" for us?

To answer this question, turn back the clock to child-hood, when we first hear external motivators. When we're children, our parents know far better than we do what's best for us. Not always, mind you, but usually. The younger we are, obviously, the less we know. The reason they tell us what to do so often is that we are truly clueless. Left to our own devices, we wouldn't get very far and most children would do only what they felt like doing because it was pleasurable: eat candy, play, make messes and not clean them up. In an emotionally healthy family, we recognize that we desper-ately need guidance from parents and other adults. We learn and feel terrific that someone is there to watch out for us and teach us about life, and we trust that what our caretakers are telling us is in our best interest.

However, for a number of reasons, the ways we're in-structed are not always phrased in the most sensitive ways. Pressed for time, Mom might say, "You have to clean your room before Grandma comes over," when what she means and often says is, "I'd like you to clean your room by the time Grandma gets here." If she insists that you *must* do something once in a while, it's no big deal. You're gener-ally okay about complying with her wishes because they're expressed fairly and reasonably. Moreover, if Mom is will-ing to hear your reaction to her request, you probably feel even more okay about it. Perhaps, you're right in the middle of doing math homework when Mom insists you tidy up your room, and you swear you'll do it by the time Grandma arrives. If Mom is fine with that, and you follow through, things are still cool.

But what if Mom is forever saying you *have* to do this and you *need* to do that, won't brook any disagreement, and never listens to how you feel about being bossed around? She gets angry if you don't instantly drop what you're doing—in this case, your math homework—and yells, "Clean up your room this very minute, or else!" You may be scared when she raises her voice and upset that your needs don't seem to matter.

Of course, every Mom and Dad have moments when they're stressed (like when *their* parents are coming for a visit!), and words may come flying out of their mouths that wound you. If parents are occasionally pushy, but fair and take your needs into account most of the time (especially if they apologize for being out of line), you understand that sometimes people get ruffled and you don't mind so much. But when you're served a constant diet of edicts that steamroll over your wants and needs, you may easily (and rightfully) build up a resentment about being pushed around by someone who's supposed to treat you better.

For individuals who grew up in households with one or both parents who were domineering and controlling, resentment usually builds over the years. Some kids react by being overly-compliant, others might be openly defiant, regardless of the consequences. Still others go the passive-aggressive route—dragging their feet to get things done, which is their way of saying, "Sure you can make me do something, but I'm going to take my own sweet time doing it. That'll show you."

For many of us, doing what *we* want and not what we're told to do becomes the most important goal in our lives, more important, in fact, than taking good care of ourselves. We see this, for example, when people won't allow their babies to be inoculated against childhood diseases because they think, against all scientific evidence, that *they* as parents should be the ones to make this decision. What's safest for the child gets lost in the shuffle when people are more attached to being the ones to make a decision than whether it's sensible or not.

Our parents often not only tell us what they think we should do but what we should and shouldn't feel. Here are some typical examples of such invalidations:

- You can't possibly be hungry. You just ate a sandwich.

- Stop telling me what you want. What about what I want?

- If it's good enough for your sister, it's good enough for you.

- You think you know what you want, but you don't.

- It's wrong to feel the way you do.

- I don't care what you think, just do what I say.

- You don't know what's best for you. I do.

I'm not out to bash parents, believe me. They have an enormously tough job and are limited by what they were taught and what was modeled for them growing up. Most are well meaning and don't realize how they're shaping you when they invalidate your needs. They are, even in their highly imperfect way, doing the best they can. I'm simply trying to explain why you may be a tad touchy about wanting what you want, and end up battling with yourself over your intentions.

My parents let me eat whatever I wanted, so how does the "shoulds" conflict apply to me?

It's true that many parents are not strict and controlling about food, but that doesn't mean they weren't rigid in other areas of life. If they didn't allow you to make your own age-appropriate choices on a regular basis, you may have gotten the message in general that what you want and need didn't matter.

Here's a great example of what I'm trying to explain. I had a client who was a competitive skier whose father oversaw her skiing career. From the time she was a small child, everything in her life revolved around skiing. Although she had a sweet, affable nature, her father relentlessly pressed her to be more interested in winning than in making friends with her fellow skiers.

In her late teens, she developed an eating disorder—binge-eating and bulimia—although eating had always been a rather *laissez-faire* occasion in her family. Growing up, she'd eaten pretty much what she wanted and didn't have to worry about gaining weight because she skied off most of her calories. Rather, her problems with food were her way of saying, "Listen up, everybody. I'm stressed. I have needs other than skiing. Why won't anyone let me do what I want and just leave me be!"

Get my point? Even if you had freedom around food growing up, if you didn't have it in other areas of your life, you may be playing out your struggle for autonomy with eating. I will say, however, in my 30-plus years of experience working with disregulated eaters, that the majority were not allowed to have their appetites guide them as they grew up, and it's no surprise that they have mixed feelings about eating, weight, and self-care. Sometimes they were "overweight" and their parents, or one parent, came down hard on them to shed pounds. Other times, their weight was normal for their age, but one parent, usually Mom, feared weight gain or hated fat, and acted in overt and subtle ways to restrict her eating. Either way, the parental message came across loud and clear, "You don't know what or how much to feed yourself," which was heard as, "You don't know what you need, but I do."

Food for Thought

In what ways did your parents or caretakers override what you wanted for yourself? How did you react—did you rebel, act out passive-aggressively, or become overly compliant? How do you feel now about people telling you what to do?

To recap, when we're children, there's no question that we need others to guide us and voice what's best for us. I want to be clear about that. We obviously cannot live and thrive without effective guidance. What throws a monkey wrench into the works is when parents denigrate or ignore our wants and needs—at any age. After all, our needs tell us who we are, and if we don't feel accepting about and confident in our wants and desires, how can we ever feel good about ourselves?

Parents messing with our appropriate needs (to be heard, seen, think, or feel for ourselves), even with the best of intentions, generally spawn a host of problems. Remember, we are totally dependent on our caretakers initially and for many, many years, putting us in a bind. Here's the clinical explanation of what happens when parents create such a dilemma for us—and it's not pretty. If we deny our needs and do what our parents want, we feel a loss of our own identity or individuality, nothing less than our sense of authentic self. The boundary between parent and child blurs and we (and our parents) don't know where they end and we begin. This dynamic, called *enmeshment*, hampers our budding individuality. By denying our needs and going along with what a parent wants, we gain their approval but lose our selfhood. We keep our connection with them, but not with ourselves.

Alternately, we may not go along with our parents and, instead, defy and pull far away from them. This dynamic, called *disengagement*, happens when we hold onto our connection to our wants and needs but, consequently, lose the love (or approval) of a parent for not doing whatever he or she wants us to do. We end up connected to our authentic selves but not to our parents.

Having to choose between attachment to our parents or to ourselves is an awful dilemma. Often, in order to survive, we choose attachment to them over us. This is why we may say "yes" to our parents, then do what we want. That way we preserve the connection to our parents and receive their approval but also get our own needs met. This is how teen-agers end up smoking or drinking behind their parents' backs, or why adults (whose parents are no longer around) wind up tip-toeing down to the refrigerator in the middle of the night to sneak a fat- and sugar-laden snack while their family sleeps.

Sadly, other harmful developments occur when, as a child, you're regularly and unfairly invalidated or unfairly overridden by an adult. One is gradually losing a keen sense of knowing what you want. It's highly distressing when someone is constantly telling you that you have no idea what you're feeling or talking about. It's a surefire way to learn to mistrust yourself. For example, I have a friend who spent most of her free time writing poems as a little girl and yearned to grow up to be a poet. Sadly, her poorly-educated mother had no idea that poetry need not rhyme and would scrawl (in red pen!) at the end of each verse her daughter presented to her, "You need a rhyme *hear*." (I kid you not about the misspelling!) My friend stopped writing poetry in high school (and to this day has an aversion to red ink) and only picked it up again as a hobby after her own children were grown. How heart-breaking is that? This is what I mean about how invalidation breaks your trust in yourself, never mind killing your spirit. Because of her mother's critiques, my friend didn't believe she had the talent to write poetry. However, I'm happy to say that she recently published a poem in a national poetry magazine!

Another problem when our needs are not validated and supported is that we don't feel worthy of even having needs. I wrote an entire book for women who put their needs last and others' first called *Nice Girls Finish Fat*, but either gender can suffer from a belief that having needs is wrong. The way this pretzel logic goes is that it's okay for others to have wants and desires but not okay for you. If you do feel or express anything that remotely smacks of having your own desires, you're being selfish or self-centered. Want to choose your own style of dressing, decide on a college or a career, have different tastes in music—no way! Of course, even nice girls and nice guys find a way around these dicta and a way to do for themselves. It's called eating.

A third derailment that happens when needs are ig- nored is called *acting out*, which is a way of non-verbally shouting to the world, "Hello, in case you haven't noticed, I have needs." The little boy who is constantly bossed at home and repeatedly bullies his schoolmates might be saying, "I'm tired of being pushed around." The middle girl in a family whose older or younger sisters get all the attention might frequently try to upstage them by being a pain in the butt to send her parents the message, "Hey, notice me. I matter too."

A final consequence of feeling invisible or unimportant is *rebellion*, which we're going to talk more about in a moment. Rebellion means doing the opposite of what is expected or wanted. Dad keeps pressuring you to make the football team, but you're not much interested in sports and would rather design computer games, so you continually skip afternoon practice until you're kicked off the team. You may do this consciously or unconsciously. Or Mom is forever on your case to look pretty and dress neatly and fashionably, so you go serious grunge or goth just to annoy and freak her out. However, in both cases, what you're really trying to express is your desperate desire to simply be guided by your own inner light.

Children develop successfully when they're given age-appropriate instruction and guidance. Toddlers may need their shoes tied for them, but you don't want to be doing that for your 14-year-old. If parents are flexible and understand effective child-rearing practices, they'll exert their power and direction only when it's necessary, then back off and be on call when their children require their help, which starts out as a great deal and dwindles down to not very much as they get older. Effective parenting keeps an eye toward eventually handing over the reins of being in charge of your life to you and, by the time you're an adult, advice should be given only when requested or, at the least, kept to a bare minimum.

Food for Thought

How connected are you to your wants, desires, and passions? Do you feel like apologizing for having needs or are you comfortable having them? Do others see you as a rebel, passive-aggressive, or someone who goes along to get along? How do you assert your needs, in appropriate and inappropriate ways?

I get this needs stuff, but how does it prevent me from taking consistently good care of myself?

Let's start with the fact that when parents validate and respect us as children and present their opinions in an appropriate way, we grow up to trust them and, subsequently, ourselves. We may not always be right, but we feel entitled to and fairly confident in our thoughts and feelings. We know they're meaningful to us and to others, and the validation we receive causes us to have faith in ourselves. It's unnecessary to go out of our way to prove that our wishes are important because we already know that and assume others do too. For the most part, it's a non-issue. We recognize that everyone has needs, and expect both to have our needs respected and to respect theirs.

When we're secure in our thoughts and feelings, we recognize that throughout life we're presented with choices, all of which have consequences. For instance, if Dad says he heard that there's a Nor'easter blowing our way and that we can go visit a friend if we want to, but he doesn't think it's wise, we consider the content of what he's saying and don't view his warning as an affront to our decision-making ability. We get the message that it's up to us whether or not to go out in the impending storm, and we're more apt to act sensibly than defiantly.

On the other hand, if you've been brought up to believe that you have the brain of a flea, my guess is that you might feel you have to prove yourself. Rather than view advice as take-it-or-leave-it information, you'll hear it as a decree and a critique of your competence. Instead of considering if someone else's opinion is valid, you'll feel as if they're trying to devalue yours. In this way, many, if not most, interactions are viewed as *interpersonal struggles* over who has the real power in your life. You're not totally sure that you do, because: 1) your parents have insisted that you're not capable of thinking for yourself, and 2) you've actually come to partially believe this.

If your family was preoccupied with who was right and wrong, my guess is that, as an adult, you have difficulty making effective decisions. Rather than focus on the information being conveyed, you get caught up in your right to do things your way or to, at the least, avoid doing things someone else's way. The fact that others dare try to impart wisdom to you overrides *what* they're actually saying.

Here's a great example of this dynamic: Many years ago, I had a male client whose wife absolutely had to have the last word on everything. According to her, nothing he ever said was right or good enough, and she was never wrong. They came to see me because they fought bitterly and constantly; days went by without their saying a civil word to each other. His cardiologist said the stress was literally killing him and referred them to me.

I saw them as a couple in the first session and knew nothing about their backgrounds, but I could have foretold what I would learn. No surprise that his mother was just like his wife. From the age of toddlerhood right through to his current mid-fifties, he was *still* trying to defend his point of view to Mom. He was angry and frustrated and had little idea what he really thought or felt—except that it was *not* going to be remotely what his wife (or mother) thought or felt.

So, let's say you're like this man and are confused about what to think or feel in numerous situations, yet also bristle instantly when told you *need to* do a certain thing. How do you think this dynamic plays out when you tell yourself that you *should* eat "normally," stay active, or take time for yourself? What plays out is that as one part of you desperately attempts to guide you toward health, another part of you sticks its fingers in its ears screaming, "No, no, no, I'm *not* going to let you tell me what to do."

You've turned what originally was an *interpersonal* struggle—between you and another person—into an *intrapsychic* struggle—between two different aspects of yourself. Without realizing it, you've adopted a way of motivating yourself that uses the same authoritarian words your parents used. Of course, you also retain the antipathy you had for being ordered around with these very words and this dynamic is what causes all the wrangling going on in your head.

When you're stuck in this rut, the truth is that you have little chance to make wise choices, but are merely playing out an old, unresolved conflict between the parental and child voices within you. There are glitches with this approach to problem solving. One is that you are no longer a child and have far better ways of making decisions than the reactionary, limited way you did way back when. Moreover, you have absolutely no chance of resolution while you're unaware of the immature, competing dynamics going on.

Please take a minute for this insight to sink in. You're not lazy or stupid and never were; you simply have mixed feelings, each one yanking you in opposite directions. Isn't finding out that you're merely conflicted a whole lot better than all the terrible names you've called yourself because of how you haven't been able to stay on track with eating and self-care? Now that you've correctly identified the problem, you can seek and find resolution.

Food for Thought

How often did your parents use words like *should* and *need to*? How often do you? What are some parental words or phrases they used that you tell yourself to this day? How have you turned an interpersonal struggle into an unconscious intrapsychic one?

How do my intrapsychic struggles play out in the food, fitness, and self-care arenas?

My guess is that you've never realized that each time you "should" on yourself, you're actively programming yourself to *not* do what you say you want to do. What a crazy paradox, huh? It turns out that the main way you learned to motivate yourself—with a host of commands—is the biggest de-motivator of all because of how you balk at being ordered about.

To be more specific, here's a sampling of the directives you probably give yourself over and over:

- I *shouldn't* eat that.
- *I have to* stop noshing while watching TV.
- I *musn't* skip breakfast cause then I'm hungry and eat junk the rest of the day.
- I *ought to* set up a schedule for going to the gym and just follow it.
- I *need to* stop procrastinating and get stuff done.

Can you feel the weighty pressure of these commands—the I-won't-take-no-for-an-answer push behind them? Do you notice how you viscerally recoil from their pushiness? I do. By using these words, you've stuck yourself smack in the middle of a struggle: the parent in you is trying to boss you in one direction and the kid in you is crossing its arms and saying, "No way! You can't make me!"

I don't want to go another round with myself, so what can I do?

Here's the problem in a nutshell. All along you've been *reacting* to that voice in your head that keeps cracking the whip and telling you what you *should* and *shouldn't* do. Or reacting to what others tell you to do. Reacting is an excellent choice when you rush to turn off the stove before the pasta water boils over. Quick thinking and automatic responses are absolutely essential when you or someone you love is in danger.

However, when you're in non-danger situations and need to think through effective strategies, you want a cool head and are better off being *responsive* than *reactive*, which means assembling information and gradually arriving at an informed decision. It also means letting go of old ways of thinking and having an adult conversation with yourself that does not include the voice of your parents or the child you used to be. When the adult you is in charge, only then can you move forward and continue making progress without backsliding. When making a decision, the adult you will assess the *content* of information without caring whose idea it is.

One of the secrets to making effective choices, ones that you'll stick with, is to express your intentions in appropriate, effective language—replacing the external motivators (*should, need to, ought to, have to, must, and am supposed* to) with internal motivators (*want, wish, desire, would like to,* and *prefer).* Can you hear how they have a very different ring to them than the commands you've been employing? Repeat aloud both sets of words and see how they make you feel. Internal motivators are from the heart and express your deepest truths. It's not that you *should* go to sleep at a reasonable hour. You *want* to get adequate sleep because of how refreshed you feel when you awaken in the morning. It's not that you *need to* stop eating junk food while watching TV. You *would like* to eat mindfully because you *wish* to be healthy, something you can't do when you're distracted by your favorite programs.

Obviously, you may have mixed feelings about taking action: you may *want* to go for a walk and also *want* to stay home where it's warm and cozy because outside it's chilly and blowy. Notice, in this phraseology, how there's not a *should* in sight! You want to walk for several reasons. It's beneficial to your mental and physical health, and your body will feel ever so good when you're done.

In this case, as in many cases, you both want to walk

and want not to walk. That's okay. *Shoulds* have nothing to do with it. With wants, you can talk about what the issues are straight from the heart and have a sane conversation between adult parts of yourself. Moreover, external motivators like *should* cause us to feel like victims, as if we have no say in shaping our lives, whereas internal motivators such as *want* empower us.

Let's say a part of you decides that you *should* start a serious exercise program. You're feeling mildly psyched, but mostly beleaguered by your decision. Dragging yourself to the gym three times a week, you remind yourself each day that you *need to* exercise and go because it's the "right" thing to do. No matter how much you push yourself, it still feels like a chore. Then things get crazy hectic on the job, and though you keep telling yourself you *ought to* exercise, the pressure at work is so great that you let yourself off the hook and give it up. You feel guilty but also relieved, because you've always hated feeling pressured to do anything. Of course, eventually the command that "I really *have to* get back to the gym" starts doing its Greek chorus thing, and soon the whole vicious cycle repeats itself.

A better approach would have been to say, "I want to go to the gym because I wish to improve my health," in which case your intention would arise from a desire to care *for* yourself because you care *about* yourself. Additionally, you might have felt fine about taking a week off from the gym until your work load settled down. Framing your thinking this way would provide two fairly equal sets of wants to work with in making a decision, and you'd either manage to find time to exercise or acknowledge that doing so would add even more stress to your life for the time being. The truth is, we end up doing what we *want*, not what we think we *should*. So, we're all better off when we phrase our intentions as preferences rather than pressures.

Trust me, the more you stop badgering yourself with *shoulds* and its brethren and start using *want* and its cousins, the sooner you'll stop rebelling against yourself. Why? Because you'll be speaking appropriately to yourself and your internal debate will be more adult. Plus, you'll have no automatic put-up-your-dukes reaction because you're being *should* on. Think of it like this: As adults, we're too old for people to be telling us what we should or shouldn't do—even ourselves!

Plus, the only thing we must do in this life is die. Everything else is optional. We may tell ourselves it isn't—that we *ought to finish our to do list*, that we *have to* marry or have children to be happy, or that we *must* lose weight for any number of reasons. Even on the little things, we may not believe we have a choice. The truth is we don't *have to* do the laundry today. We could walk around in dirty clothes, but we don't *want* to. We may feel inner pressure to do this or that, but none are mandatory. Only death is compulsory.

Food for Thought

What are the specific tasks you tell yourself you should, must, etc. do? What other external words do you use to motivate yourself? If you have mixed feelings, how could you phrase them as opposing wants? Make a list of these tasks with appropriate "want-want" language and practice expressing both sides of your feelings.

Will cooling it with the shoulds and thinking "want versus want" keep me from falling off the wagon?

Altering your language will provide substantial help in recognizing your authentic preferences and also prevent you from rebelling against yourself. But it's not the whole nine yards. There's also the issue of feeling deserving, which will be addressed in the next chapter.

For now, make it a practice to express your intentions from the heart. Listen to yourself as you think and speak, and make corrections as needed. Ask your friends or close family members to alert you to your use of external, rather than internal, motivational words. Upon awakening, make a mental note to spend the day monitoring and modifying your phrasing from self-commands to wishes. Then make sure to assess (with compassion, not judgment) how you did at the end of each day. Or do the old trick of dropping a coin or bill into a glass jar every time you find you're *shoulding* on yourself.

You'll be amazed at how quickly your phraseology will change. You won't be perfect at it, but you'll notice a more relaxed way of being with yourself within a few weeks. Moreover, you'll observe a diminished automatic backlash prompting you to engage in oppositional, unhealthy behaviors around food and exercise. Said another way, you'll see less intrapsychic in-fighting going on and will become kinder and more self-compassionate. When that happens, you can't help but make better choices.

Meet Charlotte and Her Conflict

The facts:

Shortly after retiring as a manager in a construction company, 67-year-old Charlotte came to me, as she put it pointing at her 350-pound frame, "to release some of this weight." She reported that she'd lost more than 100 pounds on several diets over the course of her lifetime only to regain "every single ounce and then some." She said that though she loved food, she really tried to eat healthfully most of the time. After I explained to her that I didn't deal with weight loss *per se*, but with learning to eat "normally," she agreed to give it a try.

The middle child of an alcoholic father and depressed mother, she noted that her two sisters and two brothers all had some kind of substance abuse problem—food, alcohol, gambling, or sex. She blamed their struggles on their violent, alcoholic father, but when I started asking questions about her childhood, she brushed me off, refusing to "dwell" on the past. It took several sessions to help Charlotte understand that her abusive father and two abusive husbands were not sequestered in the past but were actually connected to her eating problems today. Eventually Charlotte agreed to share some childhood stories, painful though they were. A milestone was when she cried telling me about her Dad punching her youngest sister so hard that he gave her kidney problems for life.

She said that her two oldest siblings stayed out of the house and away from Dad as much as possible, and both joined the military after high school. That left her, Mom, and a sister and brother in the house—fewer targets for Dad when he came home in a drunken rage. When I asked if anyone stood up to him, she laughed and said she did, that everyone else was too scared. She related one incident after another of barring her father from coming into the house by locking the door and threatening to hit him with her brother's baseball bat if he tried to enter. She also told him that if he dared strike any of them again, she'd kill him.

Although she had a career as a high-level manager after college, she had difficulty getting along with bosses, especially those she described as aggressive and controlling. After her divorces, and raising two children on her own, she went into therapy because "life just didn't seem worth living," and she was diagnosed with Attention Deficit Disorder, Seasonal Affective Disorder, and Depression. She was put on anti-depressants, which helped considerably.

Charlotte's conflict:

Although she'd smile like the sweet southern girl she was raised to be, Charlotte was one tough cookie. If I suggested getting to know some of her neighbors, she said they were busy-bodies, and she had no interest in making their acquaintance. When her doctor advised her to get more exercise, she'd yes him to death or change the subject. Moreover, she made endless to-do lists, but rarely got to check off an item until the very last minute, if at all. Although I tried to help her manage her ADD, she made very little progress getting things done.

A year into therapy, she made the connection between tuning out her parents as a child and the fact that as an adult she continued to tune out everyone else as well.

It was obvious to both of us that Charlotte was hard on herself, very hard. Every instruction she gave herself started with *should, need to, and have to,* and her tone of voice was punitive and disdainful. She might tell herself, "I should finish those tax forms. I'm stupid to have left them til the last minute." When I'd ask her to share her reaction to *shoulding* on herself this way, she'd reply with defiance, "Well, I don't want to fill out the forms, but I have to, don't I?" Poor Charlotte never cut herself any slack, but she managed to find some covertly by not doing the tasks she was ordering herself to do. This kind of self-bullying and oppositional stance filled her life, which was both sad and destructive.

The resolution:

I'd liked to tell you that Charlotte got with the program and stopped bullying herself, but that wouldn't be true. She did stop using a punitive tone and started to understand that she was just too angry to give it up. I suspect we'll have to do more work on her anger at life's unfairness before seeing more progress. The point is that it took Charlotte quite a while with me to even recognize that she was causing her own problems. And it was going to take quite a while longer to resolve them.

HOMEWORK

Write out these answers for yourself.

1. What have you learned about how you make choices?

2. What ideas or concepts were new to you?

3. Which made you feel better or more hopeful?

4. Which made you feel uncomfortable or anxious?

5. What specific actions can you take to make better choices for yourself regarding food, activity, and self-care?

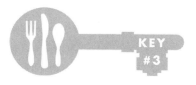

CHAPTER 6

FEEL DESERVING

(When I'm Good I'm Very, Very Good and When I'm Bad I Head for the Fridge!)

When we cherish something, we take excellent care of it. For example, is there a keepsake you treasure so much that you use the utmost care to safeguard it? I have a stuffed animal named Fluffy I've carted around with me everywhere I've moved. I don't mean to imply that I still sleep with Fluffy, although I did in my childhood. But Fluffy was such a comfort to me back then—helping me fall asleep by soaking up my childhood tears into her soft, white fur and being my best friend—and she's still in pretty respectable shape in her sixties.

We treat well what we cherish. The response is automatic, not something you have to hem and haw about, nothing you have to consider or contemplate. When you

value something, you don't lavish affection on it one moment, then kick it to the curb the next. Love is a constant, a
given.

Genuine self-care resides deep down inside and spirals
upward from a bubbling well-spring of self-love. When you
love yourself, you can't *help* but take good care of yourself. If
your default setting is, "I love and value me," then all your
actions grow from that setting. You don't need to push yourself to be kind, because you don't want to do anything *but*
treat yourself lovingly. What do you think? Does this make
sense? Take a minute to digest this idea and decide if it's
valid.

> ### Food for Thought
>
> What or whom do you love? How do you know? How
> would you describe how you act toward something you
> love versus something you don't?

I'm not saying that self-love precludes ever doing
things to cause yourself harm. No one is perfect! Being human means that there are times you'll act without thinking
and cause yourself either physical or emotional damage. You
may occasionally drink too much coffee and not be able to
sleep, or sometimes overeat yummy foods and feel stuffed,
but most of the time you monitor your coffee intake and
respect your appetite. However, if you constantly skimp on
sleep and binge on food, you are mistreating yourself and
in my mind, that self-mistreatment is what you apparently
believe you deserve. Ergo, if you think you deserve mistreat-
ment, you must not value yourself very highly.

How do I know if I love myself?

People who love themselves don't think much about it. Truly! They take it for granted and proceed accordingly. Only people who aren't sure they're worth loving need outside validation, reminders, and reinforcement. Do you just breathe or do you have to remember to do it? Most of us—barring pulmonary problems—simply breathe without thinking about the process. That's what folks who love themselves do—just love themselves without putting attention on the fact that they're doing so. This may be a new way of thinking about self-love and self-worth, so take a minute to let this truth sink in.

An outward sign of self-love is when someone cares for himself without calling his or your attention to his behavior. If you think or talk a great deal about the effort you're making to love yourself, I'd say you're on the road to self-love but not there yet. You're there when it's so integrated into your being that you have no need to think or talk about it. Rather, it oozes out of your pores and infuses all your actions.

Alternately, there are ways that lack of self-love can be recognized. One sure sign is how a person treats the question of what she *deserves*. If she keeps vacillating about whether she's entitled to something or not based on whether she deserves it, she lacks self-love. We all deserve the best in life, and people who love themselves unconditionally feel deserving all the time. Even if they mess up at work or yell at the kids occasionally, it doesn't mean they're bad people. The love they have for themselves remains untouched by these behaviors because self-love is way down deep and a work mistake or reprimanding the kids is something they *did*, not who they *are*. Get it?

Many disregulated eaters run amok with food by telling themselves something like, "I worked hard all week," therefore "I deserve that cheesecake." You betcha they deserve that cheesecake—and more. Everyone always deserves good things. But foods shouldn't be eaten or not eaten because someone feels deserving of them, but because they have a specific hunger for them. When you view questions about food not in the light of deservedness but of appetite, you get a response that is more relevant to your needs. Instead of asking, "Do I deserve a cookie," how about thinking, "Is this a food my body desires right now?" or "How will I feel after eating this food?"

Another way disregulated eaters exhibit conflicted feelings about deservedness is when they feel entitled. Clients insist, "I'm entitled to have something sweet because I came in to work early and left late," or "After taking care of the kids all day, I'm entitled to enjoy myself and eat what I want." These statements are usually said in an angry and resentful tone, as if challenging someone to deny their deservedness. People who truly feel deserving know what they're entitled to and, therefore, don't need to make an issue of it.

Even though I've spent the bulk of my professional life campaigning against all-or-nothing thinking, I'm going to make one exception here: Self- love is either there or it isn't. This dichotomy is like standing on a cliff or jumping off it. Too many disregulated eaters respond as if they're floating around in a fog when I ask them, "Do you love yourself?" or "Do you deserve the best in life?" They pause or hem and haw before answering, usually equivocally.

People who love themselves and feel deserving don't hesitate answering robustly in the affirmative. They also don't question their self-worth. On the other hand, disregulated eaters often are preoccupied with determining if they are "good" or "bad," and feel driven to act *good* (affable, kind, responsible) to counter their fears about their self-worth. In doubt about their "goodness," they're eternally seeking markers to tell them what kind of person they *really* are. Rather than having a positive default setting to begin with, they believe they must take actions to make themselves "good."

This is truly heartbreaking, because if they're not *good*, they must be *bad*. Truth is, I probably know a lot more folks with food problems than your average Joe, and I can honestly say that the majority are exceptionally caring to others, responsible, ethical, and are brimming with worthwhile attributes.

People who are self-loving don't apply terms like good or bad to themselves or wonder if they are one or the other. They understand that we are all a mixture of positive and negative traits. No one can ever be all good or all bad. The quest to be a "good" person is tilting at windmills and a waste of time and effort. Better to strive to become emotionally healthy and well-balanced, loving yourself for your pluses and minuses, because they make you uniquely you.

Life and humans are far more nuanced and complex than this kind of either-or nonsense, which reminds me of something a friend once said after we'd had a delightful lunch talking about aging, husbands, friends, former friends, and our passions. She said, "Isn't it wonderful how different we all are and how interesting that makes our lives? Wouldn't it be boring if we were all the same?" My response was to heartily agree and give three cheers to imperfection.

Food for Thought

Do you love yourself? Why? Do you deserve the best in life? Why? Are you worried about being a good person? How does this concern effect your life? Your eating and self-care?

Is loving myself the same as believing I'm lovable?

Close, but not exactly. Many disregulated eaters believe they'll only be lovable at a certain weight or when they wear a specific size. Their lovability is based on contingency. Such an individual doesn't believe she's lovable at her current size, as if being different on the outside changes who she is on the inside.

How sad that a person would pick out one arbitrary aspect of self to assign such a high, above-all-else value. Just because this distorted view comes from our culture doesn't make it any less sad. That's like saying that in a society that strongly values people who excel in math, only math geeks would be lovable (Boy, would that leave me out!), or one in which only people with green thumbs are valued, that only gardeners would be lovable. How crazy is that?

The goal for disregulated eaters is to love yourselves *unconditionally* without needing to be anything but who you are right this very minute. When self-love is *conditional* or based on contingency, there's always an "if" or "when" involved. When self-love is *unconditional*, it's based on "whatever," as in "I will love myself whatever happens." It's a permanent state of self-affection, a door that's always open, a life-time guarantee of self-satisfaction.

Lovability is not based on one or two aspects of self,

nor is it about competence, success, or talent. If it were, most of us ordinary folk would not be considered remotely lovable. Paradoxically, it's all of who you are and no single thing about you. Probably the most loved and lovable creatures on the planet are babies, and they haven't achieved anything, yet!

There must be something else involved. And there is: Being born is your ticket to lovability. Really, it's as simple as that. You are lovable because you are unique and there will never be another being quite like you. That's enough reason for you to love yourself. The truth is that you don't need to acquire self-love; all you have to do is give it to yourself. You decide you love yourself and stick with that choice *whatever* happens. And by loving yourself, you validate that you are lovable.

Many of my clients are forever seeking to know if they're lovable. If lots of people are nice to them and don't reject or abandon them, they may feel okay. However, even one person rejecting or abandoning them seems to prove that they're unlovable. That's a heck of a system for assessing lovability! Being lovable is a given, just like deservedness.

There's a psychological name for this state of shifting feelings: *unstable self-image* or *sense of self*. When you have a *stable self-image*, no matter what you do or have done, you have a balanced view of yourself. Loving yourself doesn't depend on whether people like or hate you, whether you're thrilled with your achievements or appalled by your failures. A stable sense of self brings an inner certainty and calmness that helps you stop people-pleasing or striving to be perfect. This doesn't mean you like everything about yourself (who does?) nor that you think you're terrific all the time. Rather, it gives you a soft landing place when things go wrong, as they are occasionally sure to do. You have strengths and challenges just like everyone else, good days and bad. Welcome to the human race.

> ### *Food for Thought*
>
> Write a paragraph on why you're lovable without using attributes. If you base lovability on being perfect or loved, how does that get you into emotional trouble? Do you have a stable or unstable self-image? What happens when you lose stability? What would it be like to love yourself all the time?

Where do the icky feelings about myself come from—and what's the return policy on them?

Please understand that you didn't choose your views on your lovability, deservedness, and goodness. When people were called on for wanting to have doubts and concerns about their worth, you weren't wildly waving your hand hoping to have these traits bestowed upon you. Instead, you arrived at these views through a sperm and egg uniting long ago and by being raised in a particular—unfortunately, less than optimum—environment. You are in no way, shape or form responsible for how you acquired your yucky beliefs about being substandard or defective and, in fact, you are not and never were that way.

Take a minute right now to practice loving yourself by finding that place deep inside that knows beyond a shadow of a doubt that you are completely okay and lovable. Give yourself time to pinpoint the belief and settle into it. That may take a few minutes, so relax. I don't care if all you notice initially is a fleeting flame of lovability that flickers and fades.

Right now it might be like a firefly, brightening and dimming. Just keep trying to experience loving yourself. When you've found that sweet spot, linger there a moment and enjoy!

I hope you've found that spark of self-love I'm talking about. Now it's time to wonder how you ever came to doubt your lovability.

First, let me remind you that I'm not parent-bashing. I'm simply explaining a sequence of events. I whole-heartedly believe that parents do the very best they can, and yet sometimes that's not good enough. I don't hold their shortcomings against them, because all humans are fallible creatures. Just because they become parents, doesn't confer wisdom upon them. First they're humans, *then* they're parents. Truly, there's no blame; I'm just linking up cause and effect and explaining how you got to be the way you are today.

Here goes. Children learn to love themselves in two ways: first, by what they see modeled by their parents and other family members. The case study in the last chapter about Charlotte is a telling example of what I mean. Remember Charlotte? The rebellious woman with the abusive, alcoholic father and depressed, passive mother? Do you think Charlotte's parents oozed self-love and felt deserving of good things in life? Hardly. Her mother put up with a raging, hurtful man. Had she loved and valued herself, she would have dumped him post haste. And Charlotte's Dad couldn't have felt very lovable drinking constantly and hurting his "loved ones." These are two cases of poor role modeling.

As we can see, Charlotte missed out on the first way we learn to love ourselves by having parents who model self-love. She also missed out on the second way we learn it, by *being* well loved. Here's the progression: *If they love me, I must be lovable. If they don't love me, then I must not be worthy of love.* Charlotte's mother tried to love her by keeping her out of Dad's way, but that's not much to hold onto. Her father acted as if he didn't give a fig for his children, so what was Charlotte supposed to surmise about her value from his actions?

Most parents, however, are not out and out abusive or neglectful. The majority aren't nearly as hurtful as Charlotte's, though some are like Jekyll and Hyde, depending on their mood. For example, sometimes Mom fixes healthy meals and Dad takes the kids out bike riding after dinner. Homework support is there and laughter fills the house. Until it doesn't, when Mom stops cleaning up and stays in bed all day, or Dad spends his paycheck before Mom can cash it. Parents who go from providing a safe and dependable household to absenting their obligations make it hard for children to know what to expect. They can't tell which personality Mom or Dad is going to have when they walk into a room—the nice Mom who'll go over their history homework with them or the one who'll scream for no apparent reason.

This shifting behavior is confusing for children, more disconcerting in some ways than when parents are outright abusive most of the time. Awful as that is, children can adjust because life is consistent and predictable. They know they need to keep quiet, operate below a parent's radar, and generally stay out of their way to maximize emotional and physical safety. As one client said, "When my father hit me, I knew what he was doing was wrong, that parents weren't supposed to beat their kids. But when he wouldn't talk to me for days or buy me clothes or things I needed for school, I just thought I'd done something wrong to upset him."

Parents don't mean to be erratic, but for some, rather

than respond to external cues such as their children's needs, they respond to their own internal distress. Then there are parents who go all out to take care of their children's physical needs but ignore their emotional ones. They're willing to take you to band practice, but become distant or preoccupied when you want to talk about feelings. In this way, children can come to believe that some needs are okay to have and some aren't, which translates into it's okay to care for yourself in some, but not all, ways. For, example, I had a client whose mother was constantly asking her how she felt and what was going on inside her, but would actually forget to pick her up after soccer practice. What message might my client infer from her mother's negligence?

This dynamic is called a double message: Children feel valued and not valued, cared for and not cared for and, more pointedly, loved and unloved. This situation gets even more complicated when a child is encouraged to express her needs, then is told she shouldn't have them or that she doesn't feel the way she does. Many disregulated eaters grew up with this kind of message coming at them day and night. It is translated by the child as, "You shouldn't have those needs, you are wrong." Suffice it to say that there are far more ways than outright abuse and neglect that can cause a child to feel undeserving, unloved, and unlovable.

Food for Thought

Was your parents' self-care consistently good, inconsistent, or consistently poor? What about their care for you? What messages about self-care did you learn in childhood? How do you play them out today?

What about if I believe there's something really wrong with me, like I'm defective?

When I ask clients what they mean by defective, they often hesitate and have a difficult time explaining. "There's just something wrong with me," they'll say, or, "I'm a mess and not fixable." Notice that nothing specific is offered. When I probe deeper, they may express that they were born defective, like a bad seed. The more we explore, the more confused they get about their defectiveness, which is my goal. Confusion is one of my favorite emotions, because it opens up the possibility that they're not defective or damaged after all and never were.

If you feel a vague sense of defectiveness, tell me this, Where's the evidence to prove you right? What if you're wrong, and have actually always been whole and fine? Gives you something to chew on, doesn't it? If you weren't defective and aren't now, that must mean you're just like the rest of us, a mixed bag of pros and cons—still and always lovable, deserving, and worth taking care of.

Those of you in whom the perception of a bad, damaged self is highly internalized may have to struggle to let it go. Therapy will help, as will reading books on the subject, especially about the damage that toxic parents can inflict and about how authenticity can be lost in children and regained in adulthood. If you're open to the possibility that you're okay and always have been, you'll come to believe it someday. Just don't give up the quest because there's nothing more freeing and enlivening.

> ## Food for Thought
>
> Do you feel damaged or defective? How does this erroneous perception affect your eating and self-care? Can you entertain the possibility that there's nothing wrong with you and that you've always been fine?

How will viewing myself as whole and healthy effect my eating and self-care?

There are two ways your eating and self-care can go awry. One is when you don't feel loving toward yourself. Remember: we only take care of what we value. If you don't believe you're worth a plug nickel, how much energy are you going to expend caring for yourself? If you don't care, you won't take care.

The second derailment is more subtle. If you're anything like the disregulated eaters I've known, chances are you'll take care of yourself for a while, perhaps because you feel you *should* eat healthfully and exercise, then gradually return to your more carefree and careless ways. *Careless* is an apt word here, isn't it? When you're in the mode of poor self-care you really could care less about yourself. This happens when you aren't sure how you feel about yourself and gravitate to what's familiar: self-devaluation leading to self-neglect. This happens when your default setting is shame rather than pride, when perfection and all-or-nothing thinking take precedence over simply accepting your imperfections, and when you start to feel really good about yourself and doubt that the feeling will last or that you deserve it.

The way out of this dilemma is to tolerate the initial discomfort of feeling good about yourself, sit with unfamiliar positive emotions, and refuse to give up feeling and believing you're loveable. When your default setting shifts from "defective, damaged, and unlovable" to "lovable and deserving," you're on the right track and ready to sustain effective self-care. Every fiber of your being will want to feed on healthy food, maintain your body in good working order, enjoy time relaxing, get enough sleep, and make sure you're having enough fun and pleasure. Gone will be your doubts and mixed feelings. As the Beatles sang, "All you need is love." In this case, self-love.

Meet Rick and His Conflict

The facts:

Rick was 42 years old when he came to see me, a never married tech consultant making just enough money to get by. Although he was out of shape and his doctors told him he should lose 30 pounds, he had a boyish grin that lit up his face and made me like him instantly. He explained that he was tired of "looking in the mirror and seeing my out-of-shape self," then getting into shape only to return to how I was seeing him now. "What's wrong with me? Please, tell me," he pleaded. He confessed to being lonely, but insisted that he didn't want to look for a girlfriend or apply for a full-time job, adding, "Nobody's going to want me looking like this."

Our early sessions focused mostly on his history of eating healthfully and being active through biking and walking for a few months at a time, then gradually putting less and less attention on these activities until he lost all his gains— or as he put it, "Gained all my losses." Did I mention that

he had a quick wit? He added that when he was into taking care of himself, he had his hair cut regularly and went
for monthly massages that a friend gave him at half-price,
but that these indulgences fell by the wayside as well when
he backslid. Moreover, he liked a neat and clean apartment,
but let it go when he was in a slump until he was so sick of
looking at his mess that he felt compelled to clean it up.
He was stumped about his behavior and begged me to help
him understand what he called his "psycho yo-yo pattern"
of treating himself in such a haphazard fashion.

Rick's conflict:

It didn't take long to figure out what was going on with
his see-saw behavior when Rick told me about his childhood. His father was demanding, a Navy man who ran a
tight ship. Rick's two older brothers were just like Dad, natural leaders and go-getters, whereas Rick was quiet, shy, and
had dyslexia, making school difficult for him.

Rick's mother, an artist, was exactly the opposite of his
father. She was raised in Spain in a small village and was
an easy-going, joyful woman, passionate only about her
painting. She and Rick's father would get into ear-splitting
screaming matches about how she kept the house—dirty
and messy—and for a while after a major skirmish, she
would pick up after the boys, vacuum, and have meals ready
on time. But when she became engrossed in a painting, the
boys would have to fend for themselves and the house returned to being a disaster area. Rick even wondered if his
mom's neglect went beyond artistic absorption, if this was
maybe his mother's way of getting back at his father for nag-
ging and badgering her.

When Rick's Dad was in port and at home, his focus

was on his boys and family life. When he was at sea, depending on whether or not his mother was in the midst of working on a project, Rick got anywhere from some to no attention. His brothers were out of the house a great deal, and Rick would try to help his mother cook and clean, but never felt he could keep up with his school work and the mess three boys (and his mother) made.

Rick had several issues going on which played into his on-again-off-again self-care. The first was his belief that he was the rotten apple in the barrel. So unlike his father, brothers and mother, he often wondered if he was adopted. He felt there was something very wrong with him—the dyslexia didn't help—that could never be fixed and he made only half-hearted efforts to improve because he always expected to fail. He also had unhealthy self-care models to learn from. Dad was never anything but immaculate and demanded perfection from his sons. Mom, on the other hand, had little interest in how the boys dressed, ate, or did their chores. They were lucky if she bought groceries and fixed meals. Her own self-care depended on whether she was painting or not. When she was absorbed with her art, she wouldn't shower for days or pay attention to anything else.

Rick didn't know whom to emulate. He just assumed that when he got older he'd figure it all out somehow, but never did. Sometimes he was like his dad—full steam ahead—and sometimes like his Mom, letting things go until he could stand it no longer. Moreover, Rick wasn't sure he deserved the good life. He worked for himself because he was uncertain he could keep a job working for someone else, but this meant not having the higher income he craved. He really was betwixed and betweened.

The resolution:

Once we explored what was yanking Rick one way, then the other, he could see why he had never been able to sustain progress. For all his life, he'd felt defective and undeserving and was relieved to recognize that there was never anything wrong with him that couldn't be fixed. He could see that anything less than failure was how his father and brothers operated, but that he could choose a less rigid path.

Gradually, he began to recognize how much he didn't want to be like his mother, so involved with her passion that she ignored everything else, even those she loved. He feared that if he worked for an outside company, he'd throw himself into the corporate world and never have any kind of outside life. He saw working for himself, even at a lower wage, as taking care of himself in one way, but not another. He expressed a wish to resume biking and walking. To get back into shape, he decided to return to healthful eating, while giving himself the latitude of occasional treats rather than trying to keep to a rigid diet, as he'd done before.

On the romantic front, he thought he would join an online dating service and see what happened, but try not to get seriously involved until he felt more confident and secure in himself. Down the line, he began to send out resumes to companies he thought might have the right work environment for him. Although Rick didn't feel completely solid about himself, he finally understood his self-care dilemma sufficiently enough to work on preventing it from getting in the way of consistently loving and treating himself well.

HOMEWORK

Write out these answers for yourself.

1. What did you learn about deservedness, lovability, and defectiveness in this chapter that you can use to change your eating, fitness routine, and self-care?

2. What ideas or concepts were new to you?

3. Which made you feel better or more hopeful?

4. Which made you feel uncomfortable or anxious?

5. Based on this chapter, what specific actions can you take to feel less defective and more deserving and lovable?

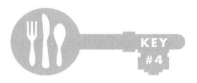

CHAPTER 7

COMFORT YOURSELF EFFECTIVELY

*(I'm Better at Licking the Bowl
than My Problems!)*

If life weren't so darned hard, you might think, *I wouldn't have this eating problem.* Well, I hate to be a downer, but you'd be wrong. Your dysfunctional eating is due to more than the stresses and strains of life. It stems from an amalgam of biology, genetics, culture, upbringing, and formative events, which create your attitude toward food and your body. This combination of factors influences how you deal with the twists and turns of life—with or without food.

Boy, does life present us with challenges. That "us," by the way, includes everyone. No one, no matter how you might idealize them, escapes life's trials and tribulations. People we love dearly die, dreams get dashed, our bodies fail us (especially as we get older—trust me!), stress gets to us, and there are times we may want to throw in the towel and say, "Okay, life, I give, you win."

The problem isn't that life goes off and does its own funky thing while we're stumbling along trying to do ours. It's the way we perceive this divergence as somehow unfair and impossible to deal with. I'm not saying you shouldn't have feelings about what happens to you. I am saying that what you *believe about* your experiences determines your reaction to it. Start from the premise that life is unfair, and you won't be disappointed!

Before moving on to talk about comfort and coping with stress and distress, let's examine beliefs that might be causing some—or even a great deal—of your problems. Although learning and practicing self-soothing and coping skills are essential to negotiating life effectively, let's not put the cart before the horse. Sure, you want to learn how to manage life without abusing food and your body, but the fact is that many of your difficulties can be eliminated by having a realistic outlook about what life dishes up.

Here's an anecdote from my clinical files to illustrate unhelpful beliefs. I had a client, Sharon, whose mother took care of all of her daughter's problems and worries growing up. Sharon would mention wanting a blue sweater, and a few days later, *voilà,* her mother would be eagerly taking several out of the box asking Sharon which one she liked best. Sharon's Mom did practically everything for her, which Sharon kind of thought was cool and also kind of resented.

No surprise that when Sharon arrived at college, she was almost totally skill-less in the life management department. She had poor study habits, was clueless how to make friends, and barely knew how to clean up the suite she shared with three other students. Over time her grades dropped, she went out less and less, and she became depressed. The one habit she practiced religiously was eating. When her room-mates went out, Sharon dug into the goodies she'd snuck into the suite.

By the skin of her teeth, Sharon did manage, with ongo-ing tutoring (paid for by Mom, of course), to finish college, but she remained depressed. Naturally, it was her mother who determined that her daughter needed help, found me, and did all the logistical work to set up an appointment. Sharon and I worked together for a number of years. Poor Sharon thought life should be easy, success should be hers merely for wanting it, friends would flock to her, and that she was a total failure if things didn't work out. We spent hours talking about how her habit of comforting herself with food and using it as a coping mechanism was based on her erroneous beliefs about life and the limited skills she had. Over time, as she gradually recognized this truth, Sharon was able to become more self-reliant. The beginning of that one-eighty was her realization that she had a faulty belief system and needed to replace it with one that was healthier and more realistic.

Food for Thought

What makes it hard to comfort yourself without food? Which beliefs might be hindering you? Which would be better beliefs for finding true comfort?

What are the best ways to manage food without stress and distress—oops, I mean manage stress and distress without food?

Rather than focus solely on learning better ways to manage stress and enhance self-soothing, it's vital for dis-regulated eaters to acknowledge and reframe the irrational beliefs that create stress and get them so agitated that it's hard to remain calm and cope appropriately. Let me lay out the kind of irrational belief system that sets up a person for intense stress and distress. Feel free to give a nod to any that speak to you because, in a moment, you'll be identifying your own belief system related to comfort and coping. Note: This exercise gives you another opportunity to be curious and self-reflective without judgment. Which of these beliefs resonate with you?

1. Life should or must be easy.
2. Feeling frustrated means I'm doing something wrong.
3. I either do things well and feel happy or do them poorly and feel terrible.
4. I need other people to provide comfort and help me cope.
5. Nothing else makes me feel better than food does.
6. I don't know how to make myself feel better without food.
7. If I don't use food to cope, I'll become dysfunctional or depressed.
8. I can't stand a lot of stress or I'm a mess.

9. I hate feeling emotionally uncomfortable or being in emotional pain.

10. When things don't go just right, it makes me feel awful.

11. I never learned to cope well, and it's too late now.

12. Nobody in my family does well with being upset, so I'm stuck being like them.

13. I'm afraid that other ways of coping won't work as well as food does.

14. I want feeling better to be instant and easy.

15. I've tried other strategies to comfort myself but they didn't work.

16. There's too much going on in my life to stop and learn new ways to comfort myself.

17. It's normal for people to turn to food when they're upset.

18. I should be able to handle my emotions myself without looking to others for help.

19. I'm ashamed of my feelings and my problems.

20. Talking about my feelings only makes me feel worse.

Recognize any of your own thinking in these beliefs? If so, not to worry, our next step is reframing—changing beliefs to make them healthy and rational. The idea is to go from holding beliefs that are limiting and based on fear to developing ones grounded in experience and evidence. These reframings will go a long way toward pointing you in the direction of coping more effectively. Feel free to put your own positive spin on the preceeding beliefs, but for

those of you who are new to the reframing process, try
these on for size:

REFRAMING BELIEFS

Change: *Life should or must be easy.*
To: *Life is not meant to be easy or simple.*

Change: *Feeling frustrated means I'm doing something wrong.*
To: *Feeling frustrated is a normal part of moving forward and I
can tolerate it just fine.*

Change: *I either do things well and feel happy or do them poorly
and feel terrible.*
To: *I feel happy that I'm putting in effort no matter what the
outcome.*

Change: *I need other people to provide comfort and help me cope.*
To: *I can cope and comfort myself.*

Change: *Nothing makes me feel better than food does.*
To: *Eating to comfort myself only makes me feel better in the moment but worse down the road.*

Change: *I don't know how to make myself feel better without
comforting myself with food.*
To: *Many things will make me feel better if I give them a chance.*

Change: *I can't stand a lot of stress or I'm a mess.*
To: *As I learn to manage stress better, I'll be fine.*

Change: *When things don't go just right, it makes me feel awful.*
To: *I can adapt and be okay when life doesn't go just right.*

Change: *I never learned to cope well, and it's too late now.*
To: *Everyone's learning some life skills in adulthood and coping and comforting are my challenge.*

Change: *Nobody in my family does well with being upset, so I'm stuck being like them.*
To: *I can learn how to deal with emotions no matter how my family handles them.*

Change: *There's too much going on in my life to stop and learn new ways to comfort myself.*
To: *New ways of comforting myself will make me feel better about whatever I'm going through.*

Change: *It's normal for people to turn to food when they're upset.*
To: *It's normal for people to turn to food occasionally when they're upset, but not to depend on it for comfort exclusively as I've been doing.*

Change: *I should be able to handle my emotions myself without looking to others for help.*
To: *Everyone can use help in dealing with some of their feelings.*

Change: *I'm ashamed of my feelings and my problems.*
To: *Upsetting feelings or problems are nothing to be ashamed of.*

Get the hang of it? Remember that these reframed beliefs are only one version out of many possibilities. There are others that might feel more right for you. Okay, I did my part. Now it's your turn. Make a list of your beliefs about comfort and coping. Don't worry for now whether they're rational or irrational and please don't fret about grammar, spelling or punctuation. Just jot down a rough list. When you think you're done, stay put for a few additional minutes and ask yourself if there's anything you left out and want to add.

Assuming there were at least a few beliefs that resonated with you, make note of them and write your reframed rational beliefs on a new list, like I did in the previous chart. Reread this list frequently—post it on your bathroom mirror, on the computer, on the fridge—especially on the fridge! Repeat it aloud whenever you get the chance. These beliefs are the foundation of learning to comfort yourself effectively without food. Yes, change is about behavior, but it's also about what you believe that leads to the actions you choose (yes, choose) to take.

Food for Thought

How did that exercise go? What feelings came up for you? Did they make you feel like eating to avoid discomfort? How else can you comfort yourself right now?

How come I instantly start thinking about food or weight when I feel crummy or am under the gun?

To help you feel a little less crazy on this subject of emotional eating, let me give you a bit of the biology and sociology that drives us toward food when we're upset. First off, it's not surprising that we seek carbohydrates when life isn't going swimmingly. When we experience emotional tension, which I'll call distress or stress, caused by internal or external pressure, our body registers emotional pain and turns to our adrenal glands, which have the evolutionary function to generate the analgesic *cortisol*. Cortisol, in turn, stimulates another brain chemical called *neuropeptide Y* that turns on and off carbohydrate cravings.

In short, stress or distress causes your body to go into defense mode to protect you from pain and ends up stimulating your appetite. Not what you'd hoped to hear, I'm sure, but that's how we've evolved. Primitive people, of course, didn't consume more carbs than their bodies needed; they were lucky to find enough to stay alive. These days, with diminished physical activity, our bodies consume more carbs than they need, particularly those high in fat, which are then converted into body fat. Moreover, some of these chemicals also make our bodies hold onto new body fat.

One more piece of information to digest. Carbs trigger another chemical reaction, one that produces *serotonin*, a neurotransmitter that relaxes us. The more tension and stress we feel, the more we drain our reserves of serotonin, which pushes our bodies to produce more. How? By eating more carbs, of course. They don't call 'em comfort foods for nothing!

Now you can understand why upset, stressed out disregulated eaters often crave carbs, specifically those high in fat and sugar. These foods *do* relax you. You haven't made it up—it's a biological fact.

The psycho-social reasons we turn to food when stressed or distressed are far simpler. First, we observe our parents head for the carbs when they're upset and follow like little ducklings. If our parents model stress-reduction-by-carb-ingestion, we're likely to follow suit. Maybe it started with grandma, who solves every problem (of hers and ours) with a box of home-made cookies. In this kind of feeling-to-food environment, no 10-year-old is likely to figure out that yoga, meditation, or mindfulness is going to be better for him in the long-run than polishing off a bag of M&Ms.

Second, we're routinely given treats to make us feel better: Have a cookie and a glass of milk and forget about your troubles, let's go to McDonalds to cheer you up. I'm not saying that an occasional sweet doesn't do the trick when you're a kid and you're down. I am saying that if you learned from childhood experience that food is the elixir to take away emotional pain, you're creating a link between the two that's going to get you into trouble down the road.

Then there's our food-oriented culture that seduces us into believing that relief for emotional discomfort comes in a bowl or refrigerated container. After all, we learn by people telling us what to do and by observing what everyone else is doing. Don't get me started on food advertisements for children on TV or the placement of high sugar and fat foods on supermarket shelves! Wouldn't it be fabulous to see TV ads for other kinds of relaxation and stress reduction as often as we see happy people eating in restaurants? Fat chance unless someone's going to make a profit from them.

Food for Thought

What's your reaction to learning more about the biological reasons you crave carbs? Does this make you feel better or worse? Which cultural factors influence you most—having been given food when you were upset as a child, parental modeling of stress-induced carb eating, the media, your friends?

If I'm scared to give up food as comfort, how will I ever learn more effective strategies?

The place to start is creating a healthy belief system. Most disregulated eaters want to throw themselves into changing their behaviors, but if you're not thinking rationally, how will your behavior ever change? *Beliefs are the foundation for transformation.* I promise that by building a healthy, rational belief system, your behaviors will be far easier to change. There's a difference between planting your garden in a trash heap or in well-fertilized soil. There, I rest my case.

Let's say that every day you read aloud your new beliefs on comfort and coping, working to internalize them, that new beliefs begin to take root, and that you're ready to put some new ideas into practice. Most disregulated eaters who are frightened of giving up food for comfort are also all-or-nothing thinkers and you might be one too, so you're going to have to do a little more shifting around in the belief department to transform your behavior.

For example, you might be thinking that because you no longer wish to rely on sweets and treats to feel better, you'll be giving them up in one fell swoop. Can you see how that might not work out so well? Because you haven't *yet* learned new skills for managing your feelings, you'll be left with nothing to calm you down and raise your spirits. Back up a bit and you'll see that this is a set-up for expecting too much of yourself too soon. Change doesn't happen overnight; no one gives up a behavior and, poof, is proficient in more effective coping the next day.

The way we learn more useful strategies is incrementally, just like we learn everything else. Oh, those baby steps, I know how frustrating they are. Believe me, I understand that you just want to be there already; but, you cannot be in the future, only the present. Your present involves learning *what* to do to avoid abusing food, never mind doing it well. So, take a deep breath and embrace the fact that you'll get better at comforting yourself without food little by little. In fact, take a moment right now to comfort yourself without food.

Close your eyes and pay attention to your breath flowing in and out. Slow your breathing and pull air down through your chest and into your belly. When you exhale, pull it up from your belly and push it out through your chest. Think of inhaling calming air and exhaling all the tension in your body. Keep doing this until you feel relaxed. Now, how about some soothing, positive self-talk to remind you that change is afoot.

It's important to recognize that you may end up using food to feel better until you practice new coping skills enough to become proficient at them. You don't have to like this fact, but you do need to accept it as truth. By accepting reality, you're untangling the knot you've tied yourself up in about comfort. Your conflict has been that you want to give up food as comfort, but fear you'll be left with nothing to soothe you. There's nothing crazy or weird about that. In fact, this conflict makes a lot of sense.

As you grow and change, you'll notice that by decreasing your use of food as a comforter and slowly increasing more effective strategies, you'll no longer feel so torn. This entire dilemma will resolve as you gain expertise with new skills and recognize that they're so effective at helping you cope that you don't *want* to return to using food to feel better. Sure, you might think about zipping by a drive-through for a burger and fries after a stressful day, but then you'll recall how terrific you felt last time you drove straight home and went for a walk instead.

An example I often use with clients is of a swimmer leaving one dock for another. Off she swims looking longingly back at the dock she's left. Frightened, back she swims and is relieved to be there, until she gazes over at the other dock where she really yearns to be. So she sets out again with more determination to get there. After enough tries, she keeps swimming until she's equidistant between the two docks. Floundering and frightened, she knows she's gone too far to return to the dock she came from and, that being the case, the only realistic choice is to swim to the other dock. Sure, she's scared, but she knows she's heading to a better place, so she sets her sights, kicks her legs, starts plowing her arms into the water, and swims off in the right direction.

Food for Thought

What non-food beliefs do you have, such as all-or-nothing thinking, discomfort feeling vulnerable, or fear of burdening others, which get in the way of using effective comfort and coping strategies?

When you want comfort, do you understand what exactly it is you're looking for? I can tell you. What you're seeking is to be re-regulated after being disregulated. It makes sense. Who wants to feel all agitated inside? No one, that's who. Emotional disregulation is a highly uncomfortable state and your desire to re-regulate is absolutely normal and natural. Much better to have your heart cease pounding so hard, for your muscles to relax, to take even breaths, and for your head to clear.

Here are some examples of events and interactions that can trigger emotional disregulation: You receive a call from your daughter's school that she's in the principal's office. You're about to move clear across the state, but the movers don't show up. You're looking forward to going out on a first date with someone you've had a crush on for months, and your boss tells you everyone has to work overtime to finish a project, no exceptions. Your dog is in intensive care at the pet hospital. Okay, you get it.

We feel well regulated when everything's copacetic and life is rolling merrily along. Disregulation occurs when emotions flare and you no longer feel in control of life. When this happens, your automatic response may be to do whatever it takes to get back on track (like eat) rather than try to understand what's happening and re-regulate more effectively. Some of our most powerful emotional surges come from current situations that trigger unpleasant memories from similar situations in the past resulting in strong emotions. For instance, say a co-worker is going on and on and you're unable to get a word in edgewise. You feel anxious and angry at the same time and may or may not recognize that this is exactly how you used to feel as a child when your father didn't listen to you.

Resolving your conflict about learning to cope and comfort yourself effectively is based on specific tactics: 1) creating a rational belief system about emotions; 2) understanding the slow, gradual nature of change which can be summed up in two words—baby steps; and, 3) recognizing your natural desire for re-regulation when you're upset. Sometimes you'll wish to deepen and explore your discomfort to understand it better, while other times you'll want to move away from intense emotion so you don't get mired in it. No one approach will work every time or in every situation.

Think of these strategies as your tool kit. When you're stressed or distressed, just open up your kit and dig around to see what's needed for your particular situation. Although it might make you feel more comfortable initially, please try not to rely on any one approach exclusively. For example, you might watch TV to take your mind off your troubles and manage not to binge eat. That might work once in awhile, but you don't want to turn into a tube boob! Learning to distract yourself from upset is a great strategy, but only if it's appropriate to a situation and only if you're choosing it from among other tactics with which you're equally comfortable. I assure you that the broader the range of strategies you have, the better your chance of not abusing food.

> ### Food for Thought
>
> Are you frightened to give up turning to food for comfort? Have you tried before? If you tried and failed, why is that? What replacement strategies did you use? What worked and what didn't? What could you do differently this time to ensure that you succeed?

What are some strategies for me to try to comfort and cope without turning to food?

As a preface, let me remind you as you try out the following approaches to always utilize kindness and compassion in the learning process. No harsh words, please. No *shoulds* and *musts*. No comparing yourself to other people or impatience with your progress. Just gently but firmly suggest to yourself to try this or that idea and notice how it works out. Remember that giving yourself comfort is not simply from the words you say, but from the tone you use saying them. So many clients talk to themselves in either a harsh, punitive voice or one that sounds distant and uncaring, like automated telephone prompts. That won't work because so much of receiving comfort is hearing a soothing inner voice. So here are some comfort tools for your tool box.

Mindfulness

Mindfulness has two parts. One is grounding yourself in the present. If you're angry at your sister for leaving you in the lurch, move out of your head and into your senses. Let those negative thoughts subside. Keep your thinking in the present and focus on what you see, smell, hear, and can touch. Becoming present and connected to your physical self will slow your heart rate and clear your mind. Breathe deeply with the intention of staying present.

The second part of mindfulness is recognizing that you're having thoughts and feelings, but that you are *not* these thoughts and feelings. As in the movie *Invasion of the Body Snatchers*, alien ideas and emotions sometimes seem to take over your being. The truth is that they're nothing more than electrical impulses. For instance, if a bear came crashing through your window and charged at you while you were fuming at your inconsiderate sister from the example above, I guarantee that you would instantly forget all about her and focus only on saving your own skin.

Thoughts come and go and are a tiny part of you that you put attention on—and can take attention off. They are not all of you. Distance yourself from upsetting thoughts or feelings by picturing them floating by like clouds. There goes one...there goes another one. In this way, the thought or feeling remains out there apart from you without *being* you. Just let it go by. If it returns, simply watch it drift off again.

Here's a great analogy. In a train station, you spend your time watching trains come and go while waiting for the right one to come along, don't you? You don't hop onto every train that opens its doors in front of you. Mindfulness is being similarly selective and not engaging with thoughts that will take you in the wrong direction. Mindfulness is very effective in calming yourself down. Will it work fantastically the first time you try it? Of course not. But it's easy to learn and, with practice, works. Practice it for at least three weeks and decide if you agree with me.

Self-soothing

Most of us know how to calm down others, even if we're not yet great at soothing ourselves. Soothing comes from a very tender part of us. When we extend ourselves to others, caring flows out in our words, tone, and gestures. We can't help but feel a tug at our hearts as we empathize with the pain of another, which generates our need to make them feel better. We don't want to feel pain (even theirs), so we do the best we can to take theirs away. We know how to soothe but rarely do it for ourselves.

We learn soothing from our parents and early care-takers. Sadly, some disregulated eaters missed out on being soothed—held, rocked, crooned to—to alleviate their upset. Some have to start from scratch and learn what it feels like to be tended to before they can comfort themselves. Our problem, explained in Chapter 6 on deservedness, is that we feel that others—but not us—deserve to be treated with kindness, caring, and compassion.

Hence, soothing flows outward toward others but not inward toward ourselves. In fact, you may need to resolve your conflicted feelings about whether you deserve caring and soothing before you're able to provide it to yourself. If you're having trouble soothing yourself adequately, it's likely that you didn't have sufficient models for it in childhood and truly don't know how, don't feel worthy of self-care, or simply haven't practiced enough.

Find ways to self-soothe every day by:

Positive Self-talk

Positive self-talk is a powerful way to self-soothe. When I hear the things that come out of the mouths of disregulated eaters, I cringe, truly I do. Aside from the *shoulds* and *musts*, there are a whole litany of unkind words and phrases that, if they were directed at me, would make me feel awful. To say them to yourself only rubs salt into your emotional wounds. When you're in emotional pain, you don't want to say to yourself: "What a jerk! You don't deserve better. See, you really are stupid! Stop whining and grow up! I knew it wouldn't work out." You get the picture. If these words and phrases are painful to hear, why on earth would you want to say them to yourself?

Negative self-talk is like slowly clawing yourself to death. You rip off one chunk of self, then another and another until there's nothing left of your positive feelings. Just because some people spoke to you like that when you were growing up is no reason to continue the carnage. Positive self-talk is the antidote to negative self-talk and reduces internal distress.

Start by listening to yourself. Much of the time, something upsets disregulated eaters and they make it worse because of what they say to themselves. Let's imagine you weren't invited to a party some friends are attending. You can rip yourself to shreds with reminders of how unpopular you are, which will make you feel worse. Or, you can remind yourself that you didn't know the host very well and can understand the omission. There'll be other parties in the future. Remember, you are what you tell yourself you are. Make a list of positive things to tell yourself—and say them!

Body approaches

I know you probably wouldn't put *crying* under the rubric of self-comfort, but sometimes when you're upset, there's nothing finer than letting the tears flow. One of the ways we suffer internal distress is from the emotional tension that builds up within us. Crying is a release (and often a relief), a way of letting loose rather than holding in (and onto) the misery. I'm a huge fan of crying and have few qualms about doing it even in front of other people. In fact, I'm kind of proud of the fact that I'm not ashamed to cry in public (most of the time). Hopefully, one day you can be more open about crying too.

Another approach to self-comfort is *deep breathing*. If you want something quicker and easier than baking up a batch of chocolate chip cookies, you can't go wrong with attending to your breath. The idea is to focus on nothing but your breathing, which means each time your mind drifts (and it will charge off elsewhere frequently), bringing it back to nothing but inhale, exhale, inhale, exhale.... What I like most about deep breathing is that it travels so well. You can be doing it in the middle of a work meeting or family gathering, where no one will be the wiser that you're tuning out external stimuli and keeping calm.

When your body is tense, a great strategy is to use *relaxation exercises* to unwind. If you know one, start practicing. It's pretty easy to go from toe to head, tensing and relaxing each muscle group and coordinating your breath to inhale relaxation and exhale bodily tension. If you don't know any exercises, buy a CD to guide you along, body part by body part, into a deeply zoned-out state. It's funny, I've heard clients say that it's hard to find the time to pop in a CD and do a relaxation exercise, but these same clients will go out in the dead of winter and drive to their local food mart for a pint of cherry vanilla ice cream! Decades ago, I was guilty of this insane pretzel logic myself. Practice relaxation every day. It's great for falling asleep at night.

Connection

A major problem for disregulated eaters who want to comfort themselves is that, while they have few skills to do so, they're also often reluctant to call on others for help. Can you see how that situation leads right to the cookie jar? If we were meant to manage on our own, I doubt there'd be so many of us living so close together on the planet. Not only do we benefit when we "Reach out and touch someone," we reap rewards when we "Reach out and are touched *by* someone." I know this is a stretch for some of you, but it's the truth. After all, you and the food aren't doing so well by yourselves, are you? Then it's time to try something—or, in this case, someone—else.

Here are some reasons disregulated eaters fail to seek comfort from others: they don't want to burden people, no one will listen or care, they feel too embarrassed (they mean ashamed), they hate feeling vulnerable, and what's the point because no one can help. This kind of unhealthy thinking is at the core of disregulated eaters' fear of giving up food for comfort. They believe that asking for comfort will weaken their already paltry self-esteem and further ruin their self-image. They're terrified of what people will think if they share frailties and vulnerabilities and seek solace—mostly they believe that others will think they're weak or crazy—and they're mortified thinking of themselves as so needy they have to ask for something like comfort, which they believe they should be able to provide for themselves.

Connecting with others is vital in order to disprove the faulty logic of the above assumptions. There is no shame in asking for help; most people are delighted to provide comfort. We all feel vulnerable at times, and sharing our vulnerability makes us feel stronger and less alone; being taken care of by others can help us in ways we cannot help ourselves. Being weak is as much a part of our humanity as being strong, receiving help is a gift not a burden. Reach out for connection—in large or small ways—to at least one person every day.

Distraction

Although I don't recommend distraction as a primary antidote for being upset, sometimes it's just what the doctor ordered. Distraction can be anything: playing computer games, taking a walk, paying bills, or gardening. The best thing that distraction does is to re-regulate your disregulated emotional system. Distraction provides relief by allowing you to focus on something outside of your inner frenzy.

You don't have to do a lot for this to happen: watch a half hour of TV, make small talk with a neighbor, or take the dog for a walk. The more you're fully involved in a distraction—mind and body—the farther away you'll be from your original agita. The more quickly you return to emotional equilibrium, the less likely you'll want to re-regulate with food you're not hungry for.

> ### Food for Thought
> Which strategies do you think will be most effective for you? Are you willing to learn some of these strategies so that you're comfortable using them rather than food?

A few more words about stress

Stress is a tricky subject, and that's why I've left it for last. Stress is a perception that brings on feelings of anxiety. What is stressful to one person might not even be a blip on someone else's radar. However, there are certain fairly universal anxiety stressors—moving to another state, entering graduate school, getting married or divorced, having surgery—which might cause you to feel a tad discombobulated. On the other hand, going to a crowded shopping mall might or might not induce stress—that is, inner tension in your body and an agitated mental state.

Many disregulated eaters cause stress by telling themselves they're overwhelmed, and they say it over and over: "I'm overwhelmed, I'm so overwhelmed...." If you keep repeating it to yourself, how do you expect to feel? What they usually mean is that they're busy and that there's some time pressure to get something, or many somethings, done. Telling yourself you're overwhelmed isn't calming, it triggers anxiety.

So stop making yourself feel stressed when you're merely busy by telling yourself, "I'm busy but will get everything done, If I don't finish my to-do list that's okay, I'm fine with what I want to get done." Beware, of course, of using words like *should* and *must* because they only make you feel more agitated. Stress is not about picking up your suit from the cleaners or ferrying the kids around. That's simply life as we know it.

To recap, troubled eaters are conflicted about giving up food for comfort because they have yet to learn better ways to do it. Although there's a natural tendency to head for the carbs in situations that generate stress or distress, self-soothing with food only creates dependence. Many disregulated eaters give a mental shriek at the thought of renouncing food for comfort, mostly because they think they have to learn how to cope without it overnight. The truth is that you'll hold onto food until you explore and practice more effective ways to emotionally regulate and re-regulate. Once you do, you won't be conflicted between food and non-food ways to comfort yourself. You'll feel happier and healthier all around, food will take up less space in your day and real estate in your mind, and you'll feel bona fide emotional comfort, perhaps for the first time in your life.

Meet Reenie and Her Conflict

The facts:

Reenie, 53 and single, was referred to me by one of the doctors at the hospital where she worked as a triage nurse in the ER. He knew her as a superb and dedicated professional and was trying to encourage her to take better care of herself, especially to watch her weight. But she always told him she was fine and he needn't worry about her. When I asked why she had come to see me, she said, "because Dr. McGill thought it was a good idea." I wondered aloud what she thought about it and she shrugged and answered, "Couldn't hurt."

Forthcoming enough with the facts of her life, Reenie barely said a word about her feelings. Most of the time she said she was fine, even when she looked as if she wasn't, which was often. She described her history with no emotion. Her father, a transplant from Ireland in his teens, died of lung cancer when she was ten and, as the oldest daughter of five children, the job of taking care of her siblings was left to her while her mother worked as a school secretary. There were days when her mother was sick with the flu and went to work anyway, and other days when her mother asked her to miss school to take care of one of her sick siblings. "It's just how things were," she said with no affect.

Reenie was surrogate mother to her brothers and sisters, treating them as if they were her own children. Her father's life insurance policy, her mother's salary, and financial support from both sides of the family helped put food on the table and a roof over their heads. Her mother had strict rules for running the house in her absence and insisted that all the children study hard. Reenie matter-of-factly recalled taking her brother to the hospital when he broke his arm and bringing her geography book with her to study for a test.

Currently she had two of her siblings living with her, "until they get on their feet," and also did her best to take care of her aged mother who was in failing health. After taking a history over a few weeks, I asked what I could help Reenie with. Shaking her head, she paused, sighed, and said she guessed I could help her with her eating. She said she knew as a nurse that her nutritional habits were "the pits" but that she couldn't seem to stop thinking about food all day. She admitted that she'd been this way as a girl: after feeding her siblings, putting them to bed, and leaving dinner in the oven for her mother, she'd sneak upstairs to eat in peace and quiet. Food, she said, with a quiver to her bottom lip, was everything to her and though she knew she was hurting herself by abusing it, she couldn't bear the thought of giving it up. During this confession was the only time I saw Reenie shed a tear, her first real emotion in our sessions.

Reenie's conflict:

What an awful dilemma for Reenie. Although she was skilled in comforting others, she had never received much comfort herself. Her mother was too tired when she got home to do much more than eat, check in, and sleep. The most she did for Reenie was make sure she did her homework and help pay for her college education. But Reenie was virtually alone, acting as a mother at age 10 when she was still a child herself. She never allowed herself to feel self-pity, fear that she couldn't manage everything, or anger at being stuck in having virtually no childhood. In fact, she never allowed herself to feel much of anything. Her coping mechanism was eating; her sole comfort was food.

The resolution:

Over time, I taught Reenie the purpose of emotions and we explored which ones she might have felt growing up and which ones she might feel now, if she allowed herself. This was slow going. Initially, Reenie had been faithful about coming weekly to therapy, but all this talk about emotions triggered a flood of them, and she started to miss sessions. So we slowed down the pace and resumed talking about how she felt about her eating. This was a subject she was comfortable discussing, her obsession with food. She would talk about it all session if I didn't re-channel her, using discussion of it as a coping mechanism to regulate her feelings in therapy as she did in life.

Finally, she felt comfortable enough to confess how helpless she felt as a child raising children, which was not far afield from how she felt every day in the ER. She admitted that she felt scared most of the time growing up, and as she became more comfortable talking about her feelings of helplessness, she was able to tackle her anger at having been robbed of her childhood and sadness about her father's premature death.

Reenie understood that she was at a crossroads: She desperately wanted to find ways other than eating to comfort herself and relax. I'll tell you, Reenie was one strong-willed woman. One day she came in and said she'd had enough and asked me to help her find better ways to comfort herself. This was a turning point in our relationship, the first time she'd asked me for help rather than just accepting it passively. She decided to enroll in a class at the hospital on mindfulness and borrowed some books of mine on the subject (remember, she was very good at studying). Sometime later, she made an appointment with the nutritionist at the hospital to help monitor her food intake.

She had successes along with times when she turned to food rather than take a walk, call a friend, or write in her journal. This was all new, unchartered territory for her. Slowly, however, these healthier activities began taking the place of eating. No stranger to hard work, Reenie knew she had embarked on a worthwhile life project, but for the first time, the project was herself.

HOMEWORK

Write out these answers for yourself.

1. What did you learn in this chapter about how to comfort yourself and cope with stress and distress without food?

2. What ideas and concepts were new to you?

3. Which made you feel better or more hopeful?

4. Which made you feel uncomfortable or anxious?

5. What specific actions can you take to comfort yourself more effectively?

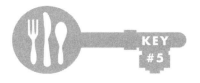

CHAPTER 8

KNOW WHAT'S ENOUGH

(Is Enough Ever Really Enough?)

I sometimes joke with clients that they suffer from an "enough disorder," because they often don't know when enough is enough in so many respects. Of course, a hallmark of disregulated eaters is pre-occupation with quantity related to food and weight, but generally the obsession about insufficiency or excess doesn't end there. Questions abound about doing enough: at work, at play, for others, and for self.

Underlying conflicts fall into two categories—*feeling deprived* (not getting enough) and *feeling inadequate* (not doing or being enough). Sometimes disregulated eaters overdo on all fronts—eating, work, parenting, cleaning...well, with just about everything. Other times, they underdo—"forget" medical appointments, quit going to the gym, withdraw socially, stop preparing healthful food, avoid chores, or cease taking care of themselves in other ways. Sound familiar?

Although you won't see the term "enough disorder" listed in any mental health manual, here are several traits that characterize it. As always, when you read through them, please don't be judgmental if you recognize yourself in any of these descriptions. The goal is to identify your "enough-ness" issues:

1. Asking others what's enough for you.

You anxiously inquire of others how they think you're doing. As if they'd know better than you would, you use their opinion to determine what's enough for you. For instance, you plan a birthday party for your six-year-old and nervously run your plans by her friends' parents, as if what they would do is what you should do.

2. Measuring yourself against others to see how you're doing.

You assess how well you've done a task by what others are doing, might do, or have done. Rather than being driven by competitive feelings, you're terrified that you might not be adequate in other eyes. Your goal isn't to be better than them, only to be "as good as" they are. An example is when you nag your friends about what they're wearing to a mutual friend's wedding. Only after you know exactly how they will be dressed do you feel comfortable selecting your attire.

3. Being preoccupied with not getting or having enough.

You're preoccupied with not receiving enough, perhaps even recognizing at the edge of consciousness that this little obsession of yours is a wee bit over the top. But you can't stop yourself: quantity and "how much" is a major fixation of yours. You notice what you and others receive and do and constantly register comparisons, most often unconsciously. This dynamic is occurring when, even as an adult, you feel a tickle of secret satisfaction that you received more holiday gifts than your siblings.

4. Bouncing from too much to too little, or from too little to too much.

Due to all-or-nothing thinking, if you feel a lack of something, you shoot to the other extreme, by trying to acquire a great deal of it. You yo-yo back and forth between scarcity and excess, underdoing and overdoing. It's exhausting to swing from one extreme to the other and still not find satisfaction, but you don't know any other way to deal with your perpetual, underlying uncertainties about what's enough. This happens when, after sitting around all winter, spring comes and you sign up for a Saturday boot camp, Zumba, and three spin classes, then two weeks into your new regime you're exhausted, can barely walk, and quit everything.

5. Experiencing intense emotions or feeling nothing.

Your emotions run from deep and intense to feeling numb in a way that makes no sense, even to you. Either you're weeping into your soup because you weren't asked to play in this year's charity golf tournament, or you act perfectly fine that your sister "forgot" to pay back the $500 she owes you and yet just went off on a cruise. Emotions have always been a bit of a puzzle to you, so you frequently go overboard with them or shut them off completely.

There's a clinical term for what I call an "enough" disorder, one which I talked about in the previous chapter: being in a state of disregulation. Think of regulation in terms of steering a small boat. If you were to yank the wheel sharply in either direction, it would swerve, list, and risk capsizing. To stay safely on an even keel, better to turn the wheel gradually and make small adjustments. This process of making incremental shifts in behavior is difficult for many disregulated eaters who, for example, often let themselves feel too empty or eat until they're too full.

Staying regulated is an ongoing issue for "disregulated" eaters, which is why I like the term better than "disordered" eaters. The word dis-regulation captures the broader dynamics. People with food problems often become easily disregulated emotionally and turn to eating to re-regulate. Mind you, we all prefer to be in equilibrium, but many folks (with or without food problems) seek inappropriate ways to re-regulate when out of balance.

Food for Thought

Which characteristics of an "enough disorder" apply to you? Do you tend to think in all-or-nothing terms? Do you ask others what's enough for you? Do your emotions swing from way too open to closed tight? Are you overly concerned with being, doing, or having enough?

How did I get this "enough" disorder? Did I catch it from someone I know?

The answer is more "yes" than "no," but perhaps not in the way you think. You didn't actually catch your "enough disorder" from your parents like you would a cold, but I'd wager that one or both of them have problems self-regulating. Maybe they have food issues like you do (which they probably call "weight" problems), or addictions to drugs, alcohol, the Internet, spending, or even work. Or they might "have to" do things to perfection or need to be in control. Maybe they follow rigid rules for just about everything for a while, then give them up for no rules at all. Perhaps they feel a need to keep busy all the time and only feel okay when they're being productive. My guess is that at least one of them engages in all-or-nothing thinking.

How do people get this way in the first place, you might wonder. Temperament and biology both play a role. By nature, we know that some folks are risk-avoiders and cautious, while others are risk-takers and comfortable at extremes. Another factor is whether or not someone has effective impulse control—that is, the ability to refrain from acting on desire alone and to calculate consequences. People who are impulsive have difficulty tolerating frustration and delaying gratification, and they often go overboard, even when doing so is not in their best interest. If they're saddled with all-or-nothing thinking, they then feel a need (or compulsion) to pull way back in the opposite direction to compensate for their excesses.

I treated a client a long time ago, a man in his early thirties, who was practically a slave to his impulses no matter what kind of trouble they got him into. He'd had a few overnight stays in jail, had contracted HIV from practicing unsafe sex, totaled I don't know how many pricey cars, and had no desire to think about the future because he was, he said, "having too much fun." It's as if his button got stuck in the "yes" position and that was that. Alternately, I've known other people who are so buttoned up that they refuse to budge from the straight and narrow, as if their "no" button was glued in place. Even talking about loosening up made them anxious. If my "fun-loving" client was too open, these folks were too closed.

Anyway, back to how you got to be the way *you* are, hurtling from one extreme to the other. By understanding what drives you, you'll be able to resolve your underlying conflicts and start to intuitively sense what's enough for you.

Before we delve more deeply into how your childhood shaped your perceptions, I wonder if you'd do me a favor. If you're wearing your "judgment cap," please take it off and set it aside. Now put on your "curiosity cap," the one that makes you interested only in gathering information and making discoveries about yourself or your past. Your curiosity cap will prevent you from making any negative assessments of what you're reading. It will allow you only to be curious about new information.

Remember, too, as you read, that I'm not out to get anyone, certainly not your parents. I'm trying to encourage you to recognize how you came to have self-regulation problems, which will help you understand and resolve your conflicts about deprivation and self-sufficiency. After all, that's the purpose of this chapter. So let's agree to be open-minded and non-judgmental about your parents, searching only for explanations and not seeking to assign blame. Fair enough?

That said, I can't stress strongly enough how much the behavior that parents model creates our childhood operating systems. Let me give you an example that's not about self-regulation, but shows all too clearly how we may follow in our parents' flawed footsteps. One day I was talking to a relative stranger in a doctors' office, while we waited for our appointments. I think that sometimes when I tell people I'm a therapist, they feel free to open up to me, which is fine because I'm ever inquisitive about human behavior. At any rate, this woman told me about her two failed marriages to powerful men and her inability to stand up to them. She was hopeful that she would pick a different kind of man now that she'd been in therapy for a few years.

When we got around to talking about her family, guess what the dynamic was between her parents. Dad was a self-made man, president of the company he'd started from scratch, tennis champ at the country club, and a large benefactor in the community, while Mom just followed along catering to his needs. This double-divorcee, their daughter, had followed exactly in her mother's footsteps. This is what humans do. We often model ourselves after our parents, for better or worse.

Food for Thought

Would you describe either of your parents as disregulated or as people who had difficulty with underdoing or overdoing or all-or-nothing thinking? How did this dynamic manifest itself? Do you have similar traits?

How do we lose touch with what's enough?

It's time to take a look at your specific fears about deprivation and insufficiency to understand where those seeds were sown. When most people consider deprivation, they immediately think about food or money. For sure, if you grew up without enough to eat, you might have serious issues with hunger and insufficiency regarding food. But how parents relate to food regarding quality and quantity also impacts our ability to judge what's enough for ourselves. Again, please keep an open mind when considering whether you've suffered deprivation in childhood. You don't have to be abused or severely neglected for an uneasy relationship with food to have developed based on feeling you haven't gotten what you wanted, needed or deserved.

For example, did you learn from your parents that there's never enough food? They may have modeled this attitude whether they were truly deprived or not. If *they* were raised in a household with a bare bones' budget, even if they had adequate financial resources raising *you*, they still may have harbored fears of not having enough. My generation, the Baby Boomers, had parents who weathered the Great Depression of the 1920s when nearly everyone worried about finances. The phrase, having a "depression" mentality, means being frugal and thrifty in the extreme, putting saving and material conservation above all else. Frugality and thrift are excellent traits, except if they're unnecessary and actually do harm instead of good, which brings us back to the *perception* or fear of deprivation.

I'm not suggesting that you delve into your family's historic and economic roots—although that might help you understand it better. My point is to help you look squarely at the attitudes your parents modeled, as well as how you experienced them. Some parents are frugal with food. They dole out small helpings and look askance if you dare to stretch your arm in the direction of seconds. This gives you the message that you'd better appear to have had enough. Well, what if your hungry body is screaming, "more" while your parents are saying, "That's it!"? Other parents eat parsimoniously themselves, maybe because they truly have a small appetite or because they're dieting. They may feed you enough, but how much food they consume influences you. While they eat sparingly, your plate is piled high with food, so you feel that you're somehow doing something wrong and they're doing it right, even without a word being spoken.

Worse, maybe you were shamed for overeating or told, "You don't need that much food. Your eyes are bigger than your stomach." This is one more message that says you don't know how much food is best for you, but someone else does. More often than not, your parents meant well. They weren't trying to starve you to death or malnourish you. Unfortunately, however, this conflict of needing to abide by or trying to please others at the expense of our own needs can plague us for a lifetime.

Some families have arbitrary rules that cause children to feel deprived. One is not being allowed to eat certain foods. A client of mine had a mother who was adamant that one container of a type of food be finished before another could be opened. For example, the Cheerios had to be gone before the Raisin Bran was opened or the pistachio ice cream needed to be finished before the strawberry swirl could be tasted.

Another type of rule involves being unable to eat a particular food because someone else wants it. I had a friend from childhood whose father was the self-appointed marshal of the refrigerator. He'd say things like, "You can't eat that. It's for your brother," or "You'd better make sure to leave some of that for your mother." Her mother had another set of guidelines: food for company. Maraschino cherries were off limits as were the "expensive" cookies she bought at the bakery, so my friend could eat only the supermarket ones. She grew up without a sense that she was entitled to choose what foods *she* craved, and when she had a family of her own, she saved the "good" stuff for them while eating the cheapest and easiest-to-fix for herself.

Subtle messages can shape your inability to determine

for yourself the right choices or amount of food to eat. Whether there really wasn't enough to go around or you were discouraged from eating whatever there was, we're talking about a lifelong conflict around food in the making.

Food for Thought

Was there a scarcity of food in your household growing up? If there was adequate food, did your parents act as if there weren't, leaving you feeling deprived? Did your parents have a "depression" mentality? What was your reaction to it? Were certain foods arbitrarily off limits or only available to particular household members or guests?

Is feeling deprived just about food and eating?

Not by a long shot! This whole subject of deprivation goes well beyond food. As I said before, it also involves perception. For example, if growing up you ate rice and beans most nights with some occasional fish or chicken thrown in, you may have felt that you had enough nourishment and never left the table hungry. But what about when you visited friends' homes for dinner and were served multiple courses and scrumptious desserts? Maybe envy caused you to want more of what your neighbors had in order to feel better about yourself. Not a food issue at all, but a self-esteem one.

You might think that actual deficits would distress us more deeply than imagined ones, but this isn't necessarily the case. That's how quirky the mind is. Maybe there were fights at the table among your siblings over who got the last scoop of mashed potatoes or the remaining cookie even when food was plentiful. These struggles made you uncomfortable around food, underscored the idea that taking what you wanted was wrong, and gave you the false impression that eating is a very serious affair with strict rules and repercussions.

I've had numerous clients who grew up with parents who were members of the food police, and swore way back then that when they became adults, they'd always eat whatever they wanted and never restrict their kids' food choices. Sometimes this attitude helps people and their children become "normal" eaters, but it can also lead to a situation without limits to what or how much can be eaten.

As you can see, there are a number of ways that conflicts around food sufficiency can be generated:

- When there's not enough to eat.

- When, although there's ample food, one or both parents act as if there's a scarcity or that it's more acceptable to eat less than more.

- When poverty means there aren't enough material goods in general.

- When there are enough foods and material goods but a scarcity and covetous mentality develops regarding what others have and you don't.

As if these possibilities aren't enough to consider, let's throw in another childhood dynamic that frequently leads to feeling deprived and inadequate later in life. This happens when parents are distant, cold, or neglectful, and children aren't sufficiently nurtured and loved. They may have plenty of food on their plates and money in their pockets, yet still sense that something essential is missing.

What is lacking comes in the form of time and attention, tenderness and compassion. This is a tall order for parents, especially if they have several children and work long hours at their jobs, yet it is what is essential to raise healthy offspring. It's not enough only to care for children physically by clothing and feeding them and putting a roof over their heads. That may be sufficient for children to survive, but not to thrive. If they are to flourish, they need a strong heart-to-heart, positive attachment to their parents, a connection in which love flows both ways.

Generations ago, parents didn't think of children as needing all of the above. In fact, they rarely thought of their offspring's emotional needs at all. In other cultures, parents believe that all children need is the material basics and to obey their elders. I've treated adults who were raised this way and, though some might think I'm being culturally insensitive, I can only say that these clients were deeply scarred by the lack of love and caring in their childhoods. Rather than see their parents as working hard to keep the family afloat, they saw indifference to their needs and wondered what was wrong with them that they received so little emotional consideration.

If their parents were tight with a dollar, they now love to shell out with their own children. If their parents made most decisions for them, they give their kids free reign over choices, even ones that are age inappropriate or to their detriment. If their parents hardly cared what they did or where they went, they hover over their kids and smother them with so much attention, their kids feel suffocated.

Here are a host of interactions that can cause children feelings of emotional deprivation:

- On several occasions, Mom forgets to pick you up

from choir practice or your softball game.

- Your parents don't help with homework or seem to care about your options after high school graduation.

- Your parents fail to show up for important school occasions such as events or parent-teacher meetings.

- You get all the hand-me-downs and nothing new for yourself.

- However hard you try in school, sports, or with your chores, your parents seem disappointed and imply you could have done more or better.

- Even if you save up money for something you want to buy, your parents say no.

- You're rarely hugged by your parents.

- Your parents often say no but won't give you a reason, insisting, "Because I'm your parent" or "Because I say so."

- Comparisons and fierce (unnecessary) competition run rampant in your family.

- Siblings make fun of your emotional needs, temperament or personality; or they make fun of people like you.

- Family members talk about you negatively as if you're not in the room.

- A parent tells you he or she wishes you'd never been born.

- Your parents say, "You won't amount to anything," "You're stupid, lazy, or inadequate", or call you unkind names or a nasty nickname.

- Your siblings get attention and praise, while you're made to feel there's something wrong with you for being different than them.

Food for Thought

Did any of the above happen to you frequently? How did you feel about it then? How do you feel about it now? Was or is feeling inadequate and deprived any part of your response?

Again, this discussion is not intended as parent-bashing. Many parents don't treat their children in the ways described above. Perhaps they learned to be great parents because theirs were loving and consistent. Or maybe they became good parents in reaction to unhappiness they experienced as children. Every parent/child relationship is different. Most parents do the best they can and are effective in some areas, but not in others.

Note that behind all the above situations is the message that you don't deserve more or better and you don't know what's right for yourself, setting you up for feeling inadequate and deprived. When you receive inadequate parenting, desiring better is a healthy response, so please think of your yearnings for what you didn't receive as positive. Feeling deprived at the parenting you received may be your way of saying, "This didn't feel right. I deserved more than you gave me emotionally." It doesn't mean, as you thought, that you wanted too much, just that what you wished for was more than your parents could give.

This sense of deprivation stays with you all the time, and that's why you're always comparing who's getting more and who's doing better, or said another way, that you're not as worthy as they are. Feeling deprived generates a sense of relentless longing and leaves you with a sense of dissatisfaction and inadequacy.

Here's a great example. An adult client and her mother were in my office learning to get along better. In the course of discussion, my client mentioned that her mother-in-law had given her a pretty nightgown as a gift—she wasn't bragging or being provocative, merely stating a fact in passing. Before the daughter had finished her sentence, her mother practically jumped off the couch and demanded, "Well, I've gotten you plenty of nightgowns, haven't I?" Can you hear the sense of inadequacy and insecurity in her words, her anguish that she hadn't measured up? The poor woman felt deprived of her daughter's recognition and value.

Another instance is keeping up with the Jones's. They buy a nice car and you feel compelled to do them one better. Your friend's son gets into Harvard while yours was accepted at Boston University (one of my alma maters), and you suddenly feel inferior. There's a piece of chocolate cake left on the serving tray at a party, and you snatch it up and eat it quickly, feeling momentarily triumphant and satisfied, but not sure why. All these actions come from a sense of not having enough.

Over time, the desire to attain satisfaction perpetually directs your attention outward. Your cravings are no longer about pleasing yourself, but involve someone else. Your quest for material goods is to quell your fear of not measuring up to your sister or best friend. Your yearning for a perfect body is to make up for all those times you didn't feel popular in school. By focusing almost obsessively on getting your share in the big world, you feel you're making up for the less-than share you had as a child. But that's something we can never make up for because we can't go back in time.

Driven by deprivation or a sense of inadequacy, which keeps you wanting more and more, you lose faith in yourself. Most people who have deprivation issues grew up with a weak sense of trusting themselves, especially if their parents were always telling them how much or how little they wanted or needed. When you don't trust yourself, your ability for self-assessment flies out the window. "How much do I want?" becomes an open-ended question. You want it all—and then some, but truth is that a dozen donuts won't generate any more satisfaction than half a dozen or half of one.

Food for Thought

How deep does your sense of deprivation run? Are you someone who feels a need to keep up with the Jones's? Do you feel "less than" when someone has more than you? Do you trust yourself to know how much food you want or need?

What if I feel as if I'm getting enough but never giving or doing enough?

You may remember that at the beginning of this chapter I said that disregulated eaters often have two conflicts: not *getting* enough, which is experienced as deprivation, and not *being or doing* enough, which is felt as inadequacy.

Disregulated eaters have these "how much?" uncertainties in many areas of their lives. They fear that however much they're doing it isn't enough and suffer guilt that they're doing less than they should. Their anxiety subsides only when they hear what an exceptional job they've done. The down side of this praise, however, is that it doesn't stick. The next time they do something, they return to their default setting of feeling as if they're not doing enough, and they're off approval-seeking again. We generally call people like this *insecure*.

It's easy to see how conflict can arise when you can't judge for yourself that what you're doing is satisfactory and acceptable. You spend a lot of time uncertain about when to start, when to stop, and how much to do in between. Here's an example: Say you've been running yourself ragged doing most of the car-pooling and are thrilled that the other parents think you're Wonder Woman. The down side is that you go home exhausted and eat cookies to boost your flagging energy. Eventually, being prone to all-or-nothing thinking, you don't just cut back a smidge on driving the kids around, but instead quit the carpool entirely.

Food for Thought

Do you generally feel as if you don't do enough? What's your typical response to that feeling? When you overdo it, do you realize it? How do you respond? Do you tend to have all-or-nothing thinking about what's enough?

Okay, I've had enough of my enough disorder. Now what?

Learning to trust yourself and feeling deserving is what sensing enoughness is all about. Remember these tips as you move forward:

1. *Look to self-regulate in small increments rather than going to extremes!*

2. *Focus on sensing enough within rather than looking outside for answers!*

3. *Don't make decisions based on entitlement!*

4. *Have faith that you can learn what's best and enough for you no matter what anyone says!*

The only way to resolve your conflict about what is or isn't enough is to develop an internal sense of sufficiency and learn to trust yourself. I know you're scared of relying on yourself because of your perceived failures in the self-trust department and may think it is impossible. But let me try to convince you that it isn't.

First, stop looking backward. Your past is not your future. You had a mindset that didn't work. Now you're learning a new one. Second, you mislabeled the problem. You thought you were deficient and it turns out you've simply based your life on mistaken interpretations of your previous experiences, especially in childhood. Third, you're discovering new ways to resolve old conflicts, which provides you with the skills and mental power to take better care of yourself.

Here's how self-trust will grow within you.

1. By looking at the world as a place of abundance, not deprivation.

This means assuming that there is plenty out there, for you, for me, for all of us—love, attention, food, success... whatever. Your belief that there's not enough has led to your need to grab onto and cling to what you can have or do, and other times to dole them out to yourself. You may have had severe limitations when you were a child because adults had all the power. You may have had fewer options or sometimes none at all. Today you're an adult and possess the power, within reason, to get what you want.

If you take off your blinders, you'll see fullness in the world. This attitude is a bit like optimists viewing a glass as half full, and pessimists seeing it as half empty. Honestly, if you don't get one job, you'll get another; and if you don't have a piece of cheesecake right now, there are other pieces of cheesecake with your name on them to be enjoyed in the future.

Typical of a deprivation mentality is what disregulated eaters call the "last supper." Better gobble it all up now because starting Monday the diet begins. Better to use the "every supper" mentality, which means that you can have foods you love every meal—even between meals. Once you know you *can* have them, you won't feel you *must* have them and won't have to gorge on them. Using self-talk that speaks to abundance rather than scarcity will calm you down when you feel panicky that you'll never have Mom's special bread pudding again or your favorite restaurant's pizza. Believing (realistically, of course) that everything is out there waiting for you will help you make choices that fulfill your cravings.

One of the biggest shifts in learning to sense sufficiency is to shake off your fears and go from deprivational thinking to abundant thinking. In the former, there's not enough of anything or everything to go around. A deprived mindset says that you must get your share now (this minute!) before it's gone or, at least, prepare yourself for being gravely disappointed when you miss out. An abundant mindset says there are many ways to meet your needs and find pleasure in life, and that the world is full of sweetness and surprise gifts made especially for you.

Imagine sitting down at a table with a large group of people while dinner is being served family style. With a scarcity mindset, you'd look at the food and anxiously fret, "I hope there's enough for me," but in a mindset of abundance, you'd think, "There's plenty of food for all of us to share, so I'll be fine." Here are some beliefs that will help you create a mindset of fullness and abundance:

- There is plenty for me and everyone.

- Missed chances often lead to better opportunities.

- I can decline food or leave it on my plate, because I know there's more where it came from.

- I can say no to material goods I desire, because I know there will be other opportunities to have them.

- My life will not fall apart if I don't get something I want.

- Life is full of goodies and pleasures all mine for the taking.

Food for Thought

Is feeling deprived an issue for you? Why? What's the difference between believing you're deprived and really being deprived? What's your plan for focusing on abundance?

2. By recognizing your uniqueness.

There is only one person in the entire universe who knows what's best for you, and that person is reading this book! Sure, your hair dresser might swear you'd look awesome with short hair; but if *you* like it long, keep it long. It doesn't matter what fabulous salaries your friends are making and how they try to steer you in particular career directions, because you're the only one who knows what work will satisfy you and how much money you need to live on. I'm not saying you should always pooh pooh others' opinions, just that no one else's voice should take the place of your own wisdom.

3. By learning from trial and error.

There is no secret method to know what's enough for you, no magic formula that the rest of the world is privy to and you're not. The way to figure out what's best is simple: by trial and error. This can be a scary prospect for people who are used to listening to others or always want to play it safe, but the truth is you're already using this method in much of your life. You make this kind of adjustment from experience, fine tuning each new action based on previous ones. If you burned the turkey last Thanksgiving, you don't want to undercook it this holiday, but hope to serve it moist, juicy and tender. You don't have to ask someone if that's the right thing to do. You sense that it is from experience.

Can you see how we spend a good part of our lives figuring out what is the right amount of something for us? What we use to come to these conclusions is trial and error—this works and that doesn't. We have an assumption, then build up evidence to test whether it's true or not. Remember that assumptions are not facts. An assumption is an idea just hanging around waiting for evidence to prove it's true or false.

I'm not giving you a science lesson here. I'm teaching you a skill that's essential to trusting yourself: Having an idea and using your experience to test out its veracity. Here's an example of how paying attention to the experience of what's enough can make or break a happy ending. Let's say that Jack and Jill have started dating and soon after, Jack decides he's *not seeing as much* of Jill as he'd like to. He asks her out *more often*, but she tells him she's busy with work, so he figures that she'd see him if she had the time. A reasonable assumption so far. But then Jill loses her job and has a great deal of free time on her hands, which she still doesn't spend with Jack.

What does experience say about Jack's assumption? If Jack is tuned into himself, he'll observe that he wants *more* from the relationship than Jill is giving and recognize that even when she has oodles of time, she's still not spending it with him. Based on that information, he can then decide if he wants to continue pursuing her (I wouldn't recommend it) or not.

Now, let's look at this story from Jill's point of view. If she were in touch with her feelings, she'd realize that she felt as if Jack wanted *too much* from her *too soon*. Had she been honest with him right from the start, she would have used her experience to see that she couldn't give Jack as *much* as he wanted.

If they both were looking at the relationship through the eyes of the scientific method—what we call trial and error—they would have seen that their idea of being a happy couple didn't test very well and that their assumption that the relationship could work was wrong. Now, what about the words I scored in italics? What's that all about? This whole scenario was about what's enough—what felt like too much for Jill was not nearly enough for Jack. Is there anyone but Jack and Jill who could have known that? Of course not. If they decided to continue to look elsewhere for potential partners, their experience with each other would become part of the trial-and-error process they must go through to find what they're looking for.

Fortunately, you can see how any assumption measures up against evidence to decide what's good for you by assessing how you feel in mind and body. That's all there is to it. Here are some assumptions you might want to take for a test drive to see if they're too much, too little, or just right:

- Going to the gym three days a week is about right for me.

- I feel satisfied without that second helping.

- Getting at least seven hours of sleep helps me eat more "normally."

- Going out every night is fun.

- I must take Mom shopping once a week or she'll be upset.

- I have plenty of clothes in my closet.

Each of these statements can be tested by you to see if they're too much, too little, or exactly what you need. Try going to the gym three days a week and see how you feel, sleep at least seven hours and notice your energy level (and how much or little you eat) the next day, have or don't have that second helping and check out your satisfaction level. Your mind and body will work together to tell you what feels right and what doesn't. Look for and build your life around the evidence of your experience, and gradually you'll develop the faith that's necessary to take care of yourself. Trust produces confidence, which produces more trust, and each reinforces the other.

Remember that sensing enoughness is not only relevant to eating. Yes, it's important to know when you feel full with food—sometimes at lunch half a sandwich will do and other times you might need a whole sandwich plus an apple—but it's equally essential to use your senses to know what you need in every aspect of life.

Food for Thought

When do you trust yourself most? Least? Do you believe that you can learn to be and stay in touch with enoughness? How willing are you to give up what you think "should" be enough and test your assumptions instead?

---

4. By feeling unconditional deservedness.

All of the changes you want to make regarding deprivation and insufficiency will come more easily if you believe you're 100% deserving 100% of the time. As I've said before, you don't need to do anything special to be deserving. It's one of the gifts of living on the planet because we are born worthwhile.

When decisions aren't based on what you believe about your worth, they're based on rational factors: Can I afford it, do I crave it, how enjoyable will it be, how will it feel and, most importantly, will it be in my long-term best interest. You make decisions based not on the question, "Am *I* worth it," but "Is *this* worth it?"

Food for Thought

What gets in the way of giving yourself unconditional love? If you could awaken tomorrow convinced that you're lovable and worthwhile, how would that affect your decisions about what is and isn't enough for you? What beliefs need to change to view yourself with positive regard all the time?

Meet Nadine and Her Conflict

The facts:

Nadine, a 42-year-old woman, sought me out after hearing one of my community talks on "normal" eating. Divorced with one son who was married and lived in another state, she was an administrative assistant in the legal department of a large construction company. She said that what resonated with her was my speaking about on-and-off self-care as a product of not feeling 100% deserving. "Making and breaking promises to myself is easy," she admitted in our first session. "It's the in-between part that's hard." She'd start a diet one day, only to abandon it a month later. When people were nice to her, she paid more attention to herself. When they weren't, she didn't care enough to do things such as brush her teeth or clean her apartment. Sometimes, she confessed, she had to push herself to feed her cat.

Taking a history, I always listen for echoes of deprivation and derailments to a client knowing when enough is enough, and there were plenty that cropped up with Nadine. Her parents' marriage split up when she was six years old, and she and her siblings ended up living with her mother. Her dad and his new wife—and soon-to-be new family—lived nearby, so Nadine got to see a good deal of him. When she stayed with him, she enjoyed more freedom, because Dad and his new wife were busy raising their young children. She enjoyed the independence and material comforts at their house, but was often lonely playing by herself and always felt less important than her step-siblings, "like an afterthought, which was pretty funny, because I was there before they were."

With her mother, life was very different. Her mother was a real estate broker who was sometimes flush and, even with child support payments, at other times nearly broke. There were days when Mom would come home holding a $3,000 check and the family would celebrate by ordering Chinese take-out and finishing every last bite. There were also days when breakfast was dry cereal, lunch was a sandwich with a thin slice of cheese in the middle, and dinner was canned spaghetti. When money was flowing, Mom lavished gifts on herself and her children. When it ran out, Mom got angry and blamed her problems on Nadine's father deserting them. Moreover, in good times her mother threw herself into being a wonderful parent, but when her bank account dwindled, so did her spirits and she withdrew from her children.

Nadine recalled never understanding what was going on and asking her siblings a lot of questions they couldn't answer: How come Dad likes his other kids better? Why can't Mom be happy all the time? Is it our fault they got divorced? All she could figure out was that they were the bad kids and Dad's new children were the good ones.

Nadine's conflict:

There was both concrete and emotional deprivation in Nadine's childhood. Not knowing from day to day whether there would be enough food made Nadine highly anxious. She ate food when it was there and went without when it wasn't. There was always plenty to eat at Dad's and that's how she found comfort for her loneliness, by over-eating when she visited him and his family. She also recalled feeling, "If I can't get his love, I'm sure going to take his food, so at least I get something."

The issue of sufficiency also came at her from different directions. Her brother said that they'd do okay if Mom put more money in the bank, but Nadine thought her mother worked hard and deserved to treat herself well when she could. To Nadine, Dad had a great deal of money and she wanted to ask if he could share more with her Mom, but didn't dare because she was certain the answer would be no. Moreover, whenever Dad did give her spending money, Nadine was never sure if she could keep it herself or she should give it to her mother, so she usually ended up holding on to half of what she received and putting the rest in the piggy bank her mother kept on the kitchen counter.

Basically, Nadine felt good about herself and life when Mom was in the money and happy. For the most part, she worked hard to earn her father and mother's love. She rarely thought about what she needed or wanted and told herself she should be satisfied with whatever she received. If she thought anything about her lovability and worth, she said, it was that she wished she'd been born into Dad's "good" family.

The resolution:

One of the initial questions I asked Nadine on this issue of deservedness was how she could explain that her natural brother and sister, whom she thought the world of, received as little as she did. Did they not deserve better, I asked. This got her thinking and led us into the first of numerous discussions about worthiness and unconditional self-love.

Down the road, she wrote a checklist of things she wanted to do for herself each day and every week—she was a compulsive list maker—and began to make more of an effort to follow through to check off items. Slowly, she began to take better care of herself, which made her feel more kindly toward herself. Then we tried something I'd not done before with a client. I asked that she stop doing all but the most important items on her list—such as going to work, paying bills, and feeding the cat—and still hold onto her positive, loving feelings about herself. This was, as expected, a tall order, and didn't go so well at first.

We also tore into Nadine beliefs about what was real and perceived deprivation, especially regarding food. She created a list of rational beliefs about abundance and practiced saying them aloud. Next, we looked at how she could sense through her body, then decide with her mind, what was enough food and not go overboard. This entailed a good deal of bodywork, and Nadine substantially slowing down the process of eating and assessing hunger after every bite. I even invited her to bring food into our sessions and share her perceptions of satiation and fullness aloud as she ate.

Then we tackled her spending habits, which were incredibly similar to her mother's: One week she could spend nearly her entire paycheck on non-essentials, then another week she'd need to borrow money from her sister to keep a minimum balance in her checking account. She went through a growth phase when, though she still bought more than necessary, she saved the receipts so she could decide what she really needed and return everything else. We both laughed at this strategy, but it helped her think through what was sufficient for her.

Nadine came in one week wondering whether she'd had enough of therapy for a while. She'd made some significant improvements with her eating and spending habits, and wanted to do other things with her free time than hang out in my office. She said she expected she'd return to therapy with me or someone else at some point, but was ready for a break. We both considered her decision as nothing less than a triumph. As long as she was developing a sense of sufficiency, it would continue to grow and spread its tendrils to other areas of her life. She now had a working experience with how to sense when enough was enough.

HOMEWORK

Write out these answers for yourself.

1. What did you learn about your conflict with knowing when enough is enough?

2. What ideas were new to you?

3. Which made you feel better or more hopeful?

4. Which made you feel uncomfortable or anxious?

5. Based on this chapter, what specific actions can you take to acquire a more accurate sense of enoughness in eating, weight, self-care?

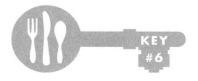

CHAPTER NINE

MANAGE INTIMACY

(Can't I Be a Super Attractive, Invisible Person?)

Intimacy and sexuality are the kinds of topics we often talk about in hushed voices. With sexuality, we sometimes even toss in a giggle or a smirk. Although the majority of us assume we're sure how we feel about being sexually and emotionally intimate, that's not always the case. It's never as easy as merely saying, "Sure I want to be loved," or "Of course, I like sex and want to be sexually attractive." *Doesn't everyone?* The truth is, sexuality and intimacy are subjects of nuanced complexity. Dollars to donuts, the broader our mish mash of unexamined feelings about love and sex are, the more likely we will act out in the food and weight arena.

I'm not saying that these are only difficult issues for disregulated eaters. Far from it. Love and sex are important in all of our lives, even if we act otherwise. Whether you've had one lover or 50, have never married or made multiple trips to the altar speaks volumes about your feelings about intimacy and sexuality. In fact, our attitudes about these subjects are extremely complicated, and that's nothing to be ashamed of.

Don't be shocked if mixed feelings arise as you read this chapter. Be curious and approach them with an open mind and heart. Remember, self-discovery is what this book is about and it's the only path to sorting out emotions. Simply notice how you feel as you read. Rather than fret about conflicting feelings surfacing, give a cheer, because they are exactly what you're trying to identify and resolve.

> ### Food for Thought
>
> How comfortable are you exploring your thoughts and feelings about intimacy? About sexuality? Do you believe there's a right and wrong way to view and experience these subjects? If so, what is the right way to view intimacy? Sexuality?

Isn't sexuality just a body thing? How'd my brain get involved?

Sexuality—our beliefs and feelings about and toward sex—are a blend of mind and body. Sure we have a physical reaction when we're attracted to someone, are aroused by foreplay, or achieve orgasm, but those goose-bumpy sensations start in our brains. In fact, none of those things that appear to happen below the neck would occur at all without all the stuff that goes on above it.

Of all the areas I discuss in this book, sexuality is perhaps the most affected by outside factors because we can't
seem to escape society's messages about it—how we should
look, what we should do in bed, what turns on a man, what
turns off a woman, what's appropriate and what's over the
line. You may think you have a mind of your own, but the
fact is you've had a whole lot of being influenced by family,
media, religion, and culture in general.

Our sexuality is purest when we're infants. Babies touch
every part of their bodies because they're exploring the world
and, since they can't get around without help, that world is
mostly their bodies. Wow, a nose; hmm, a finger; hey, a vagina. They don't differentiate between "good" and "bad" body
parts. No holds barred, they're into everything they can see
and touch, which is exactly how exploration should be. But,
as we grow into toddlerhood, neutrality toward sexual interest and expression becomes something else. That's when we
learn not just about what body parts we have, but what they
are for. For one thing, we get potty trained, which focuses
our attention (and that of others) on specific organs to the
exclusion of others. For another, we find out that we must
cover parts of our bodies that we previously comfortably ex-
posed. We don't understand the reasons for these changes;
for the most part, we just go along with the program.

And, finally, we discover that the body parts we used to
mindlessly fool around with are now taboo to fondle in public. Some children are even taught not to touch their sexual
organs when alone! So, we get the idea that anything between our neck and upper thighs is both special and strange
territory. Sadly, our innocence and neutrality about sexuality is lost by the time we're ready for school, and our pure
joy in our bodies often declines after that.

Food for Thought

Do you notice any discomfort as you're reading about sexuality? Are you aware of what's making you uncomfortable? How comfortable are you with words like penis, vagina, and orgasm?

Aside from family, who do most of our education—implicit or explicit—about sex, as children we learned about this subject, well, practically everywhere. We saw sexy images on TV and in magazines, and if we were shielded from those, we still saw them on billboards from our car seats. Grandma and Grandpa or maybe even strangers might have told us, often in passing, to pull this up or pull that down, giving us the message that some parts of us were to be censored.

Or we heard complimentary or derogatory comments about how people dressed. "My mom would never let me wear makeup like that," or "I'd love to get that t-shirt, but it's too tight across my you-know-whats." You may think this is just idle chatter, and on one level it is, but it's also the transmission of subtle messages that influence you about how to feel about your sexual self.

I recall growing up—back in the Fifties in New Jersey—and having my mother tell me not to hang out with a certain girl in my class because her shorts were too short. The instruction I was receiving was subtle but clear: Don't show off your sexual parts, because that will make boys think you like them (heaven forbid), and then you might even like them back. What my mother was saying in her own way was: Keep your sexual parts concealed so boys won't think you're advertising that you want to have sex with them and ruin your reputation, or worse, have a baby!

Out-of-wedlock pregnancy, as it used to be called, was a really (really, really) big deal in those days but not nearly as much anymore. In a novel or a movie, it used to be downright shocking if an unmarried woman had a baby. Watching *those* movies and reading *those* books shaped our attitudes about sex and sexuality. There was confusion as well. TV shows, especially sitcoms, showed a bedroom, even of a married couple, with twin beds. Couples would kiss but never go any farther. Tongue kissing was a no-no and petting would never happen.

Words describing sexual parts—like breast, penis, vagina, clitoris—were not allowed on TV or in the movies. Most things of a sexual nature were alluded to and happened off stage. Thank goodness we've gotten past those repressed times when women couldn't show their ankles because a bare leg might seduce men into thinking about sex and all hell would break loose. However, many cultures still repress women. For example, what would you infer about your sexuality if you had to wear a burka and keep your body totally covered?

It's impossible to talk about how sexual attitudes are formed without mentioning religion. Now, I know this is a touchy topic for many folks and I'll tell you right out that I consider religion, including believing that there is or is not a God, a personal issue. Be that as it may, much of society uses religion to teach morality and it definitely informs our views of sexuality. Bible teachings are used to teach right from wrong, and the sexual aspect of the self is given short thrift. Basically, virginity is highly esteemed, and sex is for marriage and creating babies. Just remember, these teachings could be interpreted as saying that we should play down sexuality no matter what our natural inclinations, and that's a powerful message. Enough said.

Well, not quite enough, because our cultural views on sexuality were founded on the Puritan ethic. Sure, today, hundreds of years after the pilgrims arrived, women have reproductive rights, censorship has become less restrictive, pornography is available with the click of a mouse, and a teenage girl now goes to school wearing less clothing than a woman wore to the beach a century ago!

But make no mistake, Puritan values still influence us and girls are still told to cover up, while at the opposite end of the spectrum is our culture's excessive, hedonistic, in-your-face sexuality. Naked, gyrating bodies are the norm on TV, while sex is talked about openly—and incessantly. This change is not necessarily bad, but it does create a clash of messages: sex is bad versus sex is good. No matter what parents or religion teach about sex, no matter what's learned in school or from peers, these wildly divergent views could make anyone's head spin. From the sexualization of fashion models and celebrities to a multi-billion dollar porn industry, you'd think we lived in a society that was totally comfortable with sexuality.

As you all know, however, this is not the case. Some folks are uncomfortable with displays of affection outside the bedroom and still use euphemisms to describe sexual organs. They still call menstruation "that time of the month" or, worse, "the curse," and refer to vaginas as "down there" and intercourse as "doing the nasty." Some even have problems with women breast-feeding in public, as if there's something too sexy about that!

Food for Thought

How have religion and culture impacted your views of sex and sexuality? What do you find conflicting in media messages on this subject? What kind of sexual conflicts does our conflicted society create in you?

You always bring up how our childhoods impact us, so aren't you going to tell us how our parents affected our sexual views?

Indeed I am. Parents are always in the mix when we're talking about how we developed our world views. So, let's dive right in—What *did* your parents think, say, and model about sex and sexuality when you were growing up? Here's what would be a healthy answer: Dad explained the birds and the bees to me, using correct anatomical language and making me believe that sex could be a beautiful, pleasurable experience. Mom read me books about my body when I was little, then talked about sex when I got older, in a way that I could tell she enjoyed it and hoped I would too. Some parents have frank, age-appropriate discussions with their children about the pill and condoms, wet dreams, masturbation, homosexuality, STDs, and pregnancy. But, truth is, most don't. Not by a long shot.

Your childhood may have consisted of nary a word said about sex or anything remotely related to it—no talks, no books, no nothing, as if sex and bodies didn't exist—from parents who rarely if ever kissed or touched in front of you. Maybe they even tsk- tsked or made negative comments when anything of a sexual nature came on a TV or refused to let you go to anything but G-rated movies. You got their message loud and clear. Or you look back at your parents' attitudes and puzzle as you remember the boring lectures you had to sit through about unwanted pregnancies and not having sex until you're married. Alternately, maybe they were openly sexual without ever saying a word about it, giving you no instruction and no idea what was appropriate or not.

Of course, being raised with messages that promote appropriate, healthy sexuality makes you less likely to be conflicted on the subject than if you received negative messages. If your parents seemed at ease with their sexuality, at home in their bodies, and tried to help you feel that way, too, you hit the jackpot. But most people are far less fortunate and receive negative messages—that sex is bad or dirty. Unfortunately, it's not so easy to shed these misconceptions when you become an adult. What's drummed into our childhood brains, especially about what our parents thought was bad and wrong, sticks with us like glue. You might want desperately to feel open and relaxed about sex, but find it difficult to shuck all its yucky or nasty connotations.

There are still other aspects of sex and sexuality that can strongly impact our adult views of it. Some parents are simply inappropriate physically and aren't cued into their children's needs about touching or kissing. There are teenagers who love to be hugged by their parents and pre-adolescents who are self-conscious and hate it. In effective parenting, Mom and Dad take cues from their children about what feels okay and what doesn't. However, many narcissistic parents are totally insensitive to and out of sync with what their children are comfortable with and pursue physical contact in order to make *themselves* feel good, even at the expense of their child's need and comfort.

Here's an example. I had a client whose generally loving father used to demand that she come over and stand by
him when she was about 12 or 13, even if she didn't want to.
He'd nag and pester until she begrudgingly inched toward
and stood in front of him with a tense body and a wary attitude. Then he'd give her a big hug and tell her how much he
loved her. She was, of course, relieved; but what a chilling,
confusing experience for a teenager.

Some children are in environments that fall short of
sexual abuse but are not quite kosher either, at least in our
culture (different cultures have different sexual mores). For
example, parents walking around half dressed or going past
the point of a hug and a kiss when their kids are beyond
latency age. At that stage, Mom feeding the baby in her bra
and panties or Dad getting in the shower with you somehow
doesn't feel right anymore. Again, emotionally healthy parents sense when their children are too old for or uncomfortable with certain behaviors. Also inappropriate activities like
touching children's sexual parts, or tickling, when a child
has aged out of this behavior or doesn't want it result in uncomfortable impressions.

Regrettably, this discussion would not be complete
without mentioning incest and sexual abuse. This behavior
is the total antithesis of teaching a child that she is in charge
of what she does with her body. If our bodies are violated
against our will—even in minor ways—we interpret that vio-
lation to mean that our bodies are not governed by us, and
it's okay for others to mistreat them. What a sad way to view
your precious self!

Non-family rape and molestation are other body boundary violations that cannot help but make healthy sexuality
confusing. Too often, even individuals who've tried to work

through the trauma of these heinous acts often experience residual, negative effects. With date rape and molestation, a person may doubt that she can trust herself to choose emotionally healthy romantic partners, be uncertain how close to allow others to get, and be confused about where the fine line between friendship and being taken advantage of is drawn.

Sexual harassment—uninvited and unwelcome advances, requests for sexual favors, and other verbal or physical misconduct that tends to create a hostile environment—can affect sexuality. It's one thing if your boss gives you a literal pat on the back for a job well done or comments that your change in hairstyle flatters you. It's quite another if he holds your hand a little longer than you're comfortable with, flirts, or makes sexually inappropriate remarks under the guise of kidding around. Moreover, sexual harassment need not come only from a superior. Colleagues can be guilty of this behavior as well. The definition of harassment is a pattern of unwanted and unsolicited inappropriateness. Even for adults who are fairly comfortable with their bodies and sexuality, this kind of behavior can be unnerving and upsetting and cause you to wonder if you're being too sensitive or are genuinely being harassed.

Food for Thought

Growing up, did you get clear or mixed messages from your parents about sex, sexuality, and your body? How about from other family members—siblings, cousins, or other adult relatives? Did you feel in charge of your body and comfortable or uncomfortable with your budding sexuality? Were there any events that were formative or influential?

How did we learn to feel conflicted about the size, shape, and weight of our bodies?

Sexuality is only one aspect of our physicality. How our bodies function and how we feel about what we see in the mirror also play a part. Since we come in all shapes and sizes—jockeys and gymnasts, quarterbacks and ballet dancers—wouldn't it be wonderful if we lived in a world in which all bodies were accepted (along with diversity in color, ethnicity, gender, and gender identity). Unfortunately, in this culture only a minority of women possess what is considered an "ideal" body—big breasts, small waist, and long legs—while the rest of us drive ourselves crazy to look like them.

Earlier, I talked about sexual violations that can happen in families, but non-sexual boundary crossing is destructive as well. This happens when parents don't accept your body as is or the way you wish it to be. For example, as a late adolescent girl, maybe you spent time lifting weights to become more muscular, which your parents found unfeminine. Or maybe they let you know they wished you were thinner. Although they may have been expressing concern for your health, their comments might have come across as a negative evaluation of your appearance. Having absorbed our cultural values equating thinness with happiness and success, parents generally mean well by their comments and are trying to improve their children's lives. However, the subtext is that there is something wrong with your body as it is. Another subtext is that appearance is more important than creativity, physical prowess, intelligence, etc. A third is that your body isn't really yours to do with what you want.

I have numerous clients who are figuratively still trying to wrest their bodies back from their parents. I once worked with a 66-year-old woman whose mother continued to ride her about carrying excess weight. This battle over who her body belonged to started when my client was a toddler, who had (unknown) food allergies that made her both bloat up from eating certain foods and also created a strong craving for them. Growing up, Mom would hide offending foods or throw them out, but my client would find them and eat them either secretly in her room or rebelliously in front of her mother. No surprise to learn that Mom was a lifetime dieter and still worked out to keep her trim figure—and at 87 was chosen as "Most Youthful Looking Senior" at her independent living facility.

Not surprisingly, my client was torn between wanting a sexual relationship and not believing that any man would want her as is, which was usually anywhere from 50 to 100 pounds over her "ideal" weight. Bright and attractive as she was, she never felt proud of her body or satisfied enough with it to have anything but brief flings, assuming that no man would want her for more than that. Not that finding a romantic relationship is a must for everyone, but this particular woman had enormous regrets that she'd wasted her life convinced that no man would ever want her "overweight" body. When I met her in therapy in her mid-sixties, she struggled mightily to break out of her body-hating mindset but, sadly, never quite could.

Another example of how conflicting feelings develop in disregulated eaters is when opposite gender parents make negative comments about their children's bodies. After all, for most of us, the way our opposite-gender parent views us sets the stage for our love relationships ever after. If a dad keeps badgering his daughter to lose weight so she'll get invited to the prom or if a mom keeps pressuring her teenage son to build some muscle because he's too skinny to ever find a girlfriend, what does that teach children about their lovability and attractiveness? We interpret these comments as saying that we're not valuable and worthy as is and wonder, "If my parents, who are supposed to love me no matter what, don't like my body, who will?"

No wonder disregulated eaters who've internalized damaging messages are confused about whether it's okay to be sexual. Here's how these conflicts play out:

Visibility or invisibility:

You might have thought I was being droll subtitling this chapter, "Can't I Be a Super Attractive, Invisible Person?" but this is a true dilemma for a large number of disregulated eaters. They yearn to be considered attractive, but then are uncomfortable with the attention they receive. Maybe it's sexual or romantic attention that frightens them, or maybe they dislike their bodies so much they would just as soon keep them hidden under layers of fat. Keeping weight on creates a buffer between what some disregulated eaters think of as their tender, vulnerable true selves and the world.

As one of my clients said with tremendous frustration, "I found out it doesn't matter if I'm fat or thin. It's still my body, and I hate it." So she would lose weight, only to seem outwardly happy, but inwardly unhappy. She'd hear praise as she toned up by dutifully going to the gym, then come home and look in the mirror and still see ugliness and grossness, until she finally gave up going. Her self-care dropped off precipitously as she lost muscle-tone and went back to non-nutritious eating.

When people have been fat, thin, and every weight in between, they can't help but be self-conscious. They think that because weight has been the be-all and end-all of *their* existence, that everyone is as focused on it as they are. They're disappointed when friends don't notice that they lost two pounds and terrified that these same people will notice that they've gained one. They want to be noticed but also don't want to be.

Sexual or not:

This culture's message is pretty much that only thin or normal weight people get to feel and be sexual, and if you're heavy, tough nuggies. People who've been fat much of their lives, especially through adolescence, may never have had a chance to try out being sexual. When they lose weight, others may make sexual advances toward them, and they may internally be at a loss of what to do, so appearing sexual— and the thought of actually *being* sexual—becomes so scary that they retreat.

If you're heavy and want to be seen as sexual, you may encounter rejection and never know if it's because of fat phobia or because of the myriad other reasons people don't click. You may believe that when you're thinner, you'll be more sexually desirable, but fear that you still won't get a second date. As a plus-size person, you can blame rejection on your weight. Better to think that than consider other flaws in your personality. In this sense, weight becomes a red herring.

Another conflict with sexuality is that you may feel sexier at a lower weight and fear becoming too desirable. Being raised to think that sex outside of marriage is dirty or wrong, you might be frightened to test yourself at a lower weight for fear that you'll enjoy being sexually active. Each of these situations can leave you riddled with conflict.

Moreover, not everyone is into sex. Some people want

to focus on career, community, self-growth, or other aspects of life, and romance is the last thing on their minds. As one of these people, life can be easier when you're at a higher weight. Prospective suitors or sexual partners leave you alone and may be happy to just be friends. That's fine with you and you're grateful to have the space to pursue other interests. But as soon as you slim down, you get hit on and feel stressed about sexual advances. So you end up either having sex because you feel you should, or figure it's not worth the trouble to fend off propositions, and put the weight back on.

One last point about sexuality and weight. Maybe you find someone who is attracted to you at a higher weight, but you're too ashamed to let him or her see your body. Fearing that your lover may sneer or laugh, or worse, reject your nakedness, you nip the relationship in the bud so you'll never have to take off your clothes and face your fears.

Food for Thought

Are you self-conscious about your body? How does your weight affect your sexuality? How does body shame affect your ability to feel or be sexual?

Okay, maybe I have some issues with sexuality, but why would I have conflicts about getting close to people if I keep my clothes on?

Intimacy seems like such a simple thing—I like you and you like me or, better yet, I love you and you love me. And we live happily ever after! Or do we? Many of us envision such a fantasy, until reality butts in and dashes our dreams or turns them into nightmares. Friendships or romances fizzle out and we're left scratching our heads, trying to figure out what went wrong.

Intimacy seems as if it should be simple, but it's anything but. Think about what it involves: opening up and showing the "real" you, accepting the authenticity of another person, trusting someone with your vulnerabilities, counting on people to be there for you, and being willing to be there for them. Is that not a tall order or what?

We think that attaining and maintaining closeness should be a snap, which leads us to believe that if we aren't close with many people, that there must be something wrong with us—we're unlovable or defective or just aren't meant to have enduring attachments in our lives. Who among us hasn't had that it's-my-fault feeling when a friendship sours or someone runs off with your heart?

Believing that we're not relationship material is enough to make us conflicted about engaging in intimacy of the romantic or non-romantic variety, but there's more going on that could create ambivalence about reaching out and touching someone. First, off, where do we learn about how to relate to people to begin with? You got it: in our family of origin. Even before we're out of the womb we're hooked into an intimate liaison with Mother. Either someone is nourishing our fetal selves with nutritious foods and relatively low stress or she's smoking and drinking, or passing on considerable stress to us.

Our primary relationship is with Mother before we can say a word or see an object. It sets the stage in many ways for our abilities to become intimate. Not that you can't overcome deficits such as Mom drinking or feeding herself—and you—poorly in utero, but it can make having relationships more difficult because of how your brain chemistry and nervous system get established.

There are a substantial number of interactions that can go right in our early family relationships. If that weren't so, many of us wouldn't be as emotionally functional as we are. Most of us grow up fairly strong and healthy, with sufficient intelligence or talent to get and keep jobs and enough interpersonal savvy to have at least a small circle of friends and some romance tossed into our lives. Fortunately, children are amazingly resilient when it comes to overcoming poor genetic loading and dysfunctional upbringings.

However, there are things that can go wrong in your childhood that make intimacy exceedingly difficult in adulthood. By understanding them, you'll get a better idea of the latent—remember, that means behind the scenes—problems that can derail intimacy and cause you to have mixed feelings about it. Let me repeat that ambivalence due to these common relational problems can be resolved so that you can develop mature attachments that are satisfying and secure. Moreover, we all have intimacy issues to a lesser or greater extent. I can't stress often enough that no one is perfect, nor should one ever hope to be (nor expect anyone they're intimate with to be) and that we're all a jumble of traits, some in decent working order and others in need of minor or major repair.

One way to view families is how *open* or *closed* they are. An *open* family system is relatively adaptable. People share their feelings appropriately and listen attentively to each other. Imagine a circle around your parents, who are in charge of your family system. They're fair, flexible, and reasonable for the most part. Now imagine a second circle around the family unit, which includes parents (or caretakers) and children. In an open system, that circle interacts with other family units frequently and comfortably—socializing, doing neighborhood and school activities. They also interact with relatives, hopefully on both sides of the family, to form an extended family, enclosed by a third, larger circle. Children get to see and form attachments to their cousins, aunts and uncles, grandparents, and maybe even great-grandparents. As well, children and parents each have relationships with their peers for fun and support. Open families are highly functional!

Then there's another kind of family, one with a *closed* system, in which many disregulated eaters were raised. Generally, this is due to major dysfunction—parental substance abuse, mental or physical illness, neglect, or sexual, emotional, or physical abuse. There are obvious and subtle unhealthy goings-on in these families, which cause them to close up tight as a fist. Parents don't invite neighbors over, frown on their children bringing friends home after school, and insist on keeping secrets about what goes on in the household—Mom's drinking, Dad's rages. Children often don't know extended family members well, and parents don't offer much information about their own histories. The closed family is an island unto itself and its motto could be us against the world. What a frightening, lonely existence for a child.

I've had many clients who barely knew their neighbors, were told next to nothing about their parents' upbringing, and never had a friend sleep over. This was normal for their household. The mindset of their parents was, "We're enough. You don't need anyone else. We'll take care of you. Other people will hurt you." Of course, that was exactly the opposite of reality, but children raised in these kinds of families didn't know that.

Closed families don't meet children's interpersonal needs and, therefore, set them up for intimacy difficulties. First off, children have far less contact with other people than they do in open systems. They simply don't have practice talking, playing, sharing emotionally, learning, or even disagreeing with others. Many are scared to have relationships with outsiders. It's easier just to keep to themselves and certainly feels safer to keep their mouths shut than to share or ask questions. Moreover, missing out on external interactions, they have no idea that there are people beyond their isolated world who would interact with them more functionally.

Children who grow up in closed-system families have difficulty being vulnerable and trusting other people. Raised with little validation, they frequently mistrust themselves. They often yearn for connections because they are lonely to the core, but their fear overwhelms them and makes reaching out or closeness unlikely. They allow themselves to make acquaintances, but rarely close friends; they might date, but the thought of having someone get to know them well enough to have a serious, ongoing relationship is terrifying beyond words. When they do date, they don't choose partners who care about them and treat them well. Rather, they hook up with partners who mistreat them as their parents did, reinforcing their belief that they're unworthy of love.

In reality, families are on a continuum from open to closed. There are some families at each end of the spectrum, but most sit somewhere along the way. They may also move in either direction as life circumstance changes—Mom gets help for her depression or Dad joins AA and stops drinking or the opposite, he falls off the wagon and goes on a bender and Mom needs to be hospitalized for suicidality. If children are lucky, the system opens up; if they're unlucky, it shuts down.

Food for Thought

Did you have a sufficient number of quality relationships within and outside your family growing up? What are your conflicts about getting close to people—and having them get close to you? How might that affect your eating, weight, body image, or self-care?

There are also two other kinds of family systems on a continuum: *parent-* and *child-centered*. In those that are *child-centered*, parents know their job is to raise happy, healthy, fulfilled children. That doesn't mean that parents don't care about their own needs; it's just that they recognize that children require a tremendous amount of attention and that, for a long time, some parental needs must be set aside. In a child-centered family, Dad doesn't say, "Well, too bad baby Linda is screaming in her crib. I'm tired, so I'm going back to sleep and let her scream her head off." Instead, Dad drags himself out of bed to see what's up with baby Linda and, if need be, quiets her down for as long as it takes. In a child-centered family, Mom doesn't park little Charlie in front of the TV for hours while she hangs out with friends in the den gabbing. Instead, she does whatever she can to entertain and relate to Charlie, even if it means missing dishing it with the gang.

You can tell a child-centered family by watching and listening to how parents and children interact. Parents ask questions, speak in a caring, but firm tone, and really want to connect with their kids. They don't go overboard surrendering to a child's wishes because this isn't good for the child either. Some people think that child-centered means giving into children's every whim. Nothing could be further from the truth; that would only create selfish, spoiled brats. Effective parents understand that children benefit from a balanced dose of no and yes. Children raised in child-centered homes internalize unconditional love from their parents and learn to love themselves, feeling valued for their own sake, not just for what or how well they do. Their parents made sure that if their children had nothing else, they at least had love.

In my experience, many disregulated eaters grew up in *parent-centered* families. Let me count the ways dysfunction occurs. The most common problem is when parents are narcissistic or self-centered. Identifiable traits in a parent-centered family are when Mom or Dad are controlling, need to be right, blame and shame others, are critical, and act as if their children are there to do for them rather than the other way around. No surprise, that parent-centered families have a great deal of substance and every other kind of abuse. Parents make sure their needs are met and their children's, not so much. Or they may not know how to love from the heart and, instead, give their children material goods, a poor substitute for meeting their emotional needs. Worse, I wince thinking of every client I've had whose parents told her that she wished she'd never been born. Talk about parent-centered! In these families, children grow up feeling like an inconvenience, not just to their parents but to everyone they meet, perhaps even to the world. How do you seek intimacy when you've never been fully loved and feel as if you shouldn't be alive?

Children raised in child-centered homes internalize unconditional love from their parents and learn to love themselves freely. Conversely, if you didn't receive sufficient love
as a child and don't know how to love yourself unconditionally, you will have to learn how now.

Food for Thought

Was your family child- or parent-centered or somewhere
in between? Was it closed or open? What family characteristics made intimacy difficult for you as an adult?
What are your major discomforts with intimacy today?

What are my sexuality and intimacy conflicts, and how does eating, weight, and self-care get caught up in them?

Here's the basic template of how your mixed feelings
might play out. Naturally a conflict consists of pros, why
you want to be close romantically or sexually, and cons,
why you don't. Remember from earlier chapters that your
pros are probably manifest, that is, in your awareness—you
yearn for companionship, enjoy a normal sex drive, and
find pleasure from being close. What's usually outside of
your awareness are the cons, what makes you uncomfortable about intimacy or sex.

Based on the above descriptions of open or closed and
child or parent-centered families, can you identify what
your fears are?

If you were raised in a *closed family,* here are just a few beliefs that would give you pause to seek intimacy whole-heartedly:

- People I don't know well can't be trusted.
- I can't let people see the real me, or they won't like me.
- It's better to keep people at a distance and show my vulnerability.
- I can't depend on others and need to rely solely on myself.
- People don't really want to hear what I have to say.
- I don't want to be stuck taking care of other people's problems.

Can you see how having any—or all—of these beliefs would bump right up against your desire for closeness? If you don't believe that another person would care about you, might that not trump your wish for intimacy? If you find trusting people scary, might that not keep you away from getting close to them? Remember, our fears usually win out over our desires.

Now let's take a look at some beliefs that might generate internal conflicts if you grew up in a *parent-centered* household. Some will overlap with the conflicts generated from living in a closed family system.

- No one really cares about me.
- People are mostly interested in themselves, not in my thoughts or feelings.
- I'm too needy and my needs are a burden to others.

• When people get to know me, they won't like me, so why bother.

• I'm safer being invisible and avoiding attachments.

• There is something really wrong with me that makes people not care about me.

No matter how much you wish for intimacy, if you hold these kinds of beliefs, they will prevent you from warming up to people and allowing them to warm up to you.

Food for Thought

How do your conflicts around intimacy or sexuality get played out with new people or friends and lovers? How do you use eating, weight, or self-care to act out these conflicts? How motivated are you to resolve them?

In particular, people who've been sexually abused as children or raped in childhood or adulthood may find it difficult to talk about what happened. Instead, they let physical and emotional distance speak for them: I'm not comfortable being touched by you, I don't want you to see my body because it stirs up too many scary feelings in me, so please, keep away and leave me alone. A perfect example is a client I had, whose brother was sexually abused by a clergyman in his pre-adolescence. My client told me how even as an adult, her brother—a sweet, kind, bright, and funny guy—could not have more than a few dates with a woman without freaking out. His sister would urge him to give someone more of a chance, but he never could. Every time a woman seemed ready for a sexual relationship, he backed off with some lame excuse. The abuse he suffered left him unable to be intimate.

Here are some questions to ask yourself:

- Do I use my weight to regulate closeness in intimate or sexual relationships?

- Might I have legitimate fears about deep emotional connections because of dysfunctions in my family growing up?

- Might I have legitimate fears about being sexual because of events in my childhood or adulthood over which I had no control?

- Do I have a habit of backing off just as I am getting close to someone for fear of being rejected or abandoned?

- Do I engage in unwanted eating rather than take risks in a relationship?

- Do I tell myself I'll have relationships when I'm thinner, when the truth is I won't allow myself to lose weight or keep it off because then I'll feel pressure to be close to people?

- Do I make excuses for avoiding close friendships or sexual relationships rather than acknowledge my fears about them?

It can be difficult to acknowledge that you aren't relationship ready. Many people who suffered earlier in their lives tell themselves they just want to put the memories behind them. What I hear far too often is, "I don't want to dwell on those things." Well, I don't want you to dwell on them either. Rather, I want you to understand what your history has done to you so you can let go of the pain and thrive in the present. However, none of us can run away from our experiences. We can make peace with the past, but only if we're willing to deal with the pain we suffered.

The first step is to look at what holds you back from having the kinds of relationships you want. Recognize that anyone can have mixed feelings about love and sex, and it's never too late to resolve your conflicts about your physical or emotional self. The longer you wait, the longer you will remain in a tug of war with your body and mind, abusing food and battling with the scale.

Start by looking at your beliefs to understand your feelings behind them. What experiences caused your fears? Recognize that life is different today and make your beliefs more appropriate to the adult empowered you. Take some small risks in the intimacy or sexuality arena to gain confidence. You don't have to be bound to the past or your interpretation of it. That was then and this is now.

Meet Jordana and Her Conflict

The facts:

Jordana came to see me because, she said, she'd tried everything else to help her lose those "damned last 10 pounds." She confessed that sometimes it was more than 10, but never more than 20, and it was driving her crazy that she couldn't get and stay at the weight she wanted. Her problem was typical: she'd eat "normally" for a while and lose weight and feel great, then out of the blue would gradually return to unhealthy eating habits and put the pounds right back on.

At 33, she was relatively happy in her life, raising two girls as a single mom after her divorce, and enjoying a job as a pharmaceutical rep. She simply didn't understand why she couldn't get a handle on her eating and weight. "Like, duh," she said to me once, "I can take care of my kids alone and bring in the bucks, but I can't eat right. I don't get it."

Her father was a successful trial lawyer who reveled in his near celebrity status and always encouraged her to make the most of herself. A no-nonsense man, he always had to be right. Her mother wrote children's books, and was highly critical of most things Jordana did. An only child, Jordana worked hard to please them both, hoping that might make them happy and end their frequent bickering.

Her own marriage had lasted seven years, ending when Jordana discovered that her husband was having an affair. Talk of how his adultery had devastated her emotionally led to her admitting that she'd always thought her father had had affairs and assumed that her mother suspected this as well. In fact, she wondered if that wasn't the underlying source of much of their discontent and squabbling.

Discussing her father's possible unfaithfulness triggered memories of him often kissing and hugging her when she did something well, but being cold and distant when she failed. As daddy's little girl, she lived for his attention but, equally, was often made uncomfortable by it. He'd tickle her and wouldn't stop until she screamed for her mother to make him leave her alone. Then, as Jordana stood there, her parents would argue about her mother's need for quiet to write and her father's accusations that he'd married a cold fish. Later, her mother would blame Jordana for pestering her father and throwing herself at him.

Jordana, attractive and popular, had dated a great deal before she met her ex-husband. Thinking back, she realized how much like her father he was: as a successful lobbyist, he traveled around the country and was what she called a "fair weather" father to the girls. Moreover, he was frequently on Jordana's case to lose weight. He was far more amorous with her when she was thinner than when she'd put on a few pounds, which upset Jordana and put more self-pressure on her to slim down.

In spite of her disappointing marriage, Jordana pushed herself to find another husband, partially because she felt it was what society expected of her, but more so because she wanted her daughters to have a father around. She dated as much as she could with her busy schedule, but told me she didn't think there was "anyone worthwhile out there." She complained that the men she liked never called her back and the ones who liked her were uninteresting and unattractive.

Jordana's conflict:

There were a number of conflicts which Jordana and I uncovered. The first was that she didn't trust men—no surprise! As we mined the subject of love and lovers, she admitted that she both wanted to get serious and didn't. She feared finding another man like her ex (and her father) and said she couldn't bear being cheated on again. Because she only allowed herself to date when her weight was at its lowest, putting on a few pounds was keeping her safe not only from the dating scene, but also from having to seriously consider potential dates as possible mates.

The more we talked about her parents' marriage, the more Jordana recognized what a mess it had been. Most of the time they'd either avoided each other or shared mutual disdain. Jordana guessed she'd rather remain single than endure what her parents had called marriage. She believed she was a better parent than either of hers had been, because she tried very hard to put her daughters' needs first, and worried that a new man might not. Moreover, she considered how even a terrific man entering their lives might disturb the relationship she had with her girls.

One session, I raised the idea that Jordana's father tickling her mercilessly might have affected her feelings about who controls her body. When the subject came up, Jordana was at first quiet, then shared how frightened she'd been of her father when he lost control. She said she never felt threatened by him sexually, but that there was a quality to his "fooling around with her" that made her physically uneasy. She thought that this was perhaps at the root of her weight loss and weight gain, a way of saying, *If I let a man get close to me, I'll lose being in charge of my body.*

The resolution:

By the time we laid out how possible reasons involving intimacy and sexuality were likely preventing Jordana from keeping off "those last 10 pounds," she was no longer so hard on herself. She could clearly see that she didn't lack self-discipline and wasn't a hopeless case, but was trying to take care of herself in the only way she knew how.

I gave her books to read about how we sometimes regulate intimacy through our size and appearance, and we discussed her conflicts nearly every session. Jordana was determined to resolve her ambivalence because she didn't want to accidentally visit them on her daughters. She also decided to stop dating for a while until she felt free and clear of her mixed feelings, which happened over the course of a few months. When she ended therapy, she not only had a better understanding of her ambivalence about sexuality and intimacy, but also a deeper awareness of how unconscious conflicts could get in the way of reaching her goals in many areas.

HOMEWORK

Write out these answers for yourself.

1. What did you learn about your intimacy or sexuality conflicts?

2. What ideas and concepts were new to you?

3. Which made you feel better or more hopeful?

4. Which made you feel uncomfortable or anxious?

5. What specific actions can you take to become more comfortable sexually, romantically, and interpersonally?

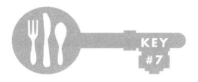

CHAPTER TEN

DEVELOP A HEALTHY IDENTITY

(If I Say Goodbye to My Identity, Will It Miss Me?)

Who are you? Of course, this is a tricky question to answer. Most of us respond by saying what we do— "I'm a social worker," or whatever our job is. But that tells us only "*What* we are" rather than "*Who* we are" which is larger, more nebulous, and requires more reflection and description.

In this chapter when I ask "Who are you?" I'm inquiring about your identity. I'm asking not only about who other people think you are, but also about the person you perceive yourself to be and the "you" that you project out into the world. Most of us carry our identity around with us as easily as a wallet in a back pocket: We know it's there and pull it out often enough but don't think much about it. Identity is *who we are* even when we're not thinking about it.

For our purpose here, identity is what you think about yourself that makes you *you*—thoughts, convictions, aspirations, fears and doubts. I'm speaking of the version of yourself that you send out into the world in conscious or unconscious ways. We all can recognize different character types: the woman whose every utterance and action aims to proclaim, "I am brilliant, special, and a force to be reckoned with," the absent-minded guy who's always forgetting his keys or misplacing theater tickets, sticklers who are overly attached to detail and see the world as a series of dotted I's and crossed T's, bad boy or girl celebrities, and dare-devils who fancy themselves invincible.

Many people are woefully unaware of how they come across. Some would be horrified if they knew, and others would deny the truth with their last dying breath. The average person doesn't arise in the morning and decide to project one particular identity onto the world—today I'll show the world how brave, selfish, cantankerous, or what an airhead, I am. Rather, they simply do whatever they do because it's who they think they are.

Mind you, by identity I don't mean striding into a job interview with a professional demeanor, a smile on your face, and your head held high. Or exhibiting your best manners when you're having your first dinner with your fiancé's parents. These are intentional ways we present ourselves to enhance our lives, and we can turn them on and off at will.

Some of us may feel stuck with our identity. Although, we may want to change our thoughts, feelings and behavior, we may consider our identity as fixed and permanent. For others, identity is something we create, because that's the person we wish to be. Some people succeed at crafting a public identity that's far different than their personal one, while others believe they are someone they're not.

This reminds me of a woman I knew decades ago who was pleasant, low-key, and fairly conventional, in no way exceptional or dramatic. Yet she mentioned off-handedly one day that she viewed herself as Auntie Mame. For those of you who don't recall the Broadway musical and movie with this title, Auntie Mame was quite a character, a free-spirited, larger-than-life woman who would stand out in any crowd. I never understood how this ordinary woman could see herself that way, but that was the identity she wished to project in the world.

Food for Thought

Name and describe some identities projected by your friends, family members, colleagues, or public figures. How about people who aim to project a particular identity—say, ladies' man, femme fatale, good ole boy, or intellectual—but don't exactly make the grade?

How do we acquire our identities, and can I exchange mine for one I like better?

By now you probably know that most of who we are is a product of our genes and socialization. We cannot separate one from the other. Babies who are exceptionally finicky and fussy may get treated more gingerly, which shapes how they might view themselves as they grow up. They might think, *I'm treated with extra care, so maybe I'm delicate or fragile and should be cautious in life.* Highly curious and adventurous toddlers may be given carte blanche to explore their world and grow into adults who push limits in sports, academics, or the creative arts. This process begins with genes that get passed down from parents, and is then shaped by these very same parents and other caretakers to form our identity. The day-by-day and minute-by-minute interactions we have with our environment mold the brain in a process called pruning.

When you're an infant and Mom or Dad talk to you a great deal and respond to your gurgles and giggles to create a conversation, you're being pruned in the direction of vocalization. When they rough-house with you and teach you athletics—to throw a ball, swing a bat, swim, or ride a bike—your brain is being pruned in the direction of physical coordination. Ditto music, sensitivity to nature, taking risks, and the gazillion other traits that make us who we are.

Also, remember that for some of us, due to genetics, acquiring various traits is either a snap or an ordeal. If your parents were tennis champs and dragged you onto the court as soon as you could hold a racquet, you had a good chance of picking up the game and excelling at it. Or hating it! If they challenged your assertions and made you defend your opinions at the dinner table, you're probably reasonably proficient at holding your own in a disagreement. Alternately, if your parents smoked, drank, sat around watching TV while munching on unhealthy snacks, your brain might have gotten pruned in the direction of passivity, mindlessness, and impulsivity.

Of course, other people shape our identities as well. One of my clients was a dancer who traveled with a national company as a youngster. Her chaperone aunt stuck to her like glue to make sure she practiced, put dance above all else, and, even at a young age, knew how to behave professionally in the public arena. Simply by sheer number of contact hours, her identity was more influenced by her aunt than by her parents.

Most everyone you come in contact with frequently helps to shape your identity—your babysitter who fires up your imagination by reading you fairy tale after fairy tale; your best friend's parents who invite you to their beach house every summer with the rest of their fun-loving clan, which goes such a long way toward teaching you how to let loose and get along with others; or the high school drama coach who casts you in a musical and convinces your parents to give you voice lessons. Of course, you can also be influenced by not-so-helpful people—your uncle who molests you and says he'll deny it if you tell your parents; your school chums who relentlessly tease you about your height, weight or other physical features; foster parents who took you in only for the money and never had a kind word to say.

As if parents, family members, and other adults aren't enough to impact our burgeoning personas, events can have tremendous influence on our lives—a brother dying of childhood leukemia; your family losing their home and belongings in a hurricane; your mom becoming paralyzed in a boating accident when you were 10; receiving a scholarship to a prestigious college; having a genius of a sister. There's no end to events that are formative to our identities, not to mention cultural, racial, religious, and other influences, which strongly shape who we are and how we are preceived.

Food for Thought

How did the following shape your identity: Your parents? Other adults? Events?

How does my identity play out in eating, weight or self-care?

Here are some identity conflicts that disregulated eaters often transmit through how they eat (healthfully or unhealthfully), what they weigh (within or outside of a healthy range), and how they take care of themselves (consistently well or poorly). A reminder that poor self-care is exhibited by inadequate or inconsistent hygiene, unsanitary and chaotic house-keeping, and engaging in unhealthy habits that harm body or mind. A word of caution however. If this descriptions fits you and you're experiencing a surge of guilt, shame or distress, please let go of these feelings. They will only hinder learning about yourself and improving your life. If this is who you are now, that's okay. You're on a path of new learning and change, so don't get hung up on who you have been.

Take a deep breath and find that place in your heart that is open, curious, and looking forward to discovering new things about yourself to improve your eating and your life. Ready? Okay, here are the identity conflicts that may plague disregulated eaters.

• *Without an eating problem, carrying excess weight, or exhibiting poor self-care, how will I protect myself from people seeing my other problems?*

There are several ways that this issue manifests itself. I've had numerous clients who had physical or mental conditions they were embarrassed about. A few were ashamed of having bipolar disorder and of the medication they took for it, Lithium, which upped their weight. Rather than acknowledge their mental problems and need for medication, they were more comfortable being seen as a fat person or overeater. I've also had clients who were taking weight-promoting steroids for serious medical conditions that they were uncomfortable talking about. For example, they feared their employers might let them go if they had any idea of the gravity of their illness. By overeating, they masked their medication-induced weight gains, therefore shielding their medical condition as well, and remained simply fat so that no one ever knew how seriously ill they were.

Now that might not make sense to you, but it was one of the ways they coped with the shame of not feeling normal. This is a more frequent occurrence than you might imagine. When I worked at the methadone clinic, I learned quickly that addicts would rather be seen, and see themselves, as drug-dependent than as people who were "mentally ill" with anxiety, depression, or PTSD.

- *Without an eating problem, carrying excess weight, or poor self-care, how will people know that I've suffered or am suffering?*

A former client of mine was in what she described as a "very good place" in her life. She had a terrific job and she and her partner of many decades had just bought a lovely house together, but she still ate emotionally on and off. She'd eat "normally" for a while and start to lose weight, then slowly put it back on. She was frustrated, disappointed in herself, and angry that she just couldn't seem to be good to herself for more than a few weeks at a time. A survivor of childhood sexual abuse as well as having grown up in a wildly dysfunctional family, one day she jokingly said to me, "My weight is like my scarlet letter. You know, to show the world that I'm fragile, so you better be good to me."

This telling comment was the key to unlocking her battle with her body based on a conflict she didn't even know she had. A strong part of her identity was as a survivor of sexual abuse. She had just begun to talk about it without breaking down crying and had only recently had her first massage because being touched had previously triggered abuse flashbacks. As is true with many abuse survivors, she felt that giving up this part of her identity would somehow invalidate what happened and was like wrenching a vital piece of self from her. Although it was painful to recognize the abuse, it was also painful to think about letting go of it as a dominant part of her identity.

Strange as it may sound, my client felt that her obesity was a way to show the world that she had suffered, as if to say, "Do you think I'd choose to be this size? I can't help it. I suffered greatly as a child and these layers of fat are proof." As we talked about other ways she could let people know her history—she ended up joining a survivors' support group— much of her emotional eating stopped. She also realized that she was highly conflicted about her identity: Was she a normal person now or was she still damaged and different? This was a conflict she needed to resolve, weight concerns and eating problems aside.

Acknowledging how identity may have morphed into a physical manifestation of suffering paves the way for moving toward a sense of now being as normal as anyone else.

Another kind of identity conflict involves current suffering. This happens a great deal within couples where one partner, usually the woman, feels unhappy and victimized. Although she wants to lose weight and be happy and healthy, her weight is her way of saying, "See, see, how miserable I am. Look what he does to me. If he treated me better, I wouldn't look this way." Of course, her perception is mistaken. Biology aside, she's made herself the way she is, and her weight is her way of getting her message out. Maybe she's afraid to admit how unhappy she is to friends or her partner. Maybe she's terrified of being alone. Whichever, she may fear speaking about her misery, so she puts it on display instead. Mostly she's ambivalent about the identity she wants to project: happy or unhappy, helpless or empowered, victim or survivor. By keeping weight on, she doesn't have to confront the truth or choose one identity over the other.

Food for Thought

Might you be using your eating, weight or self-care behaviors to send the world a message about your state of mind or identity? Do you use your size or having an eating problem to "cover" other medical or mental issues you may have? If you're someone who endures or has endured a great deal of trauma, are you attached to an identity of sufferer, victim, or "not normal" person?

• *Without an eating problem, carrying excess weight, or exhibiting poor self-care, how will people know that I'm special and need attention?*

When I was getting my bachelor's degree in elementary education, I recall being taught that children sometimes act out to call attention to themselves and that if teachers—and parents—simply would ignore the child's antics, they would stop. Well, I'm not sure that's always true, but it brings to mind how we may try in all the wrong ways to gain attention. Sadly, some people will do anything to shine a spotlight on themselves—speak loudly, boast, commandeer conversations about what *they* want to talk about, and show off.

The disregulated eaters I've worked with are exactly the opposite. They back off from being the center of attention, while encouraging others to shine. Many are self-effacing and seem more comfortable in the background than the foreground. However, to greater or lesser extent, we all enjoy feeling special and deserving of attention. Some people get it by flaunting their bodies, others by becoming emaciated, and yet others by putting on weight. Now, I'm not saying that carrying excess pounds is always attention-seeking behavior. Not at all. I am saying that for folks who find it difficult to express their craving for attention, being outside the weight range norm may be one way of getting it.

Unfortunately, the attention received in this culture when you're heavy is generally negative. Folks who are overweight are often seen as lacking in self-control or self-discipline, lazy, or even incompetent. No news to you. Not a whit of this is true, of course. Alternately, they are given "helpful" attention for their "weight problem" by friends, family, health practitioners, and even people they barely know. I've heard clients tell of being in a store shopping for clothes when someone will casually come up to them and start touting the amazing new diet they're on. Or of doctors spending more time encouraging them to lose weight than discussing the health concern they come in the door with. Or family visits in which clients' eating and weight become the central topic of conversation. Yuck, how awful!

The underlying, generally unconscious conflict some plus-size people have is this: *I would like some attention but I don't believe I deserve it.* When we're wholeheartedly convinced that we're deserving of love and attention, we enjoy receiving praise and recognition, and even the spotlight once in a while. If people go overboard with compliments, sure, we might become a bit twitchy, but we take it in stride. Unlike narcissists and folks who are highly self-centered, we don't go out of our way to seek attention, but when it comes our way for a job well done, we appreciate and enjoy the kudos.

Because so many disregulated eaters are uncomfortable with praise and attention, they and their need for acclaim or approval are often hidden and overlooked. This puts them in the position of yearning for positive reactions while feeling ashamed of their yearnings, and therefore being unable to accept the kind words that come their way. Instead, they settle for the attention they get for their perceived "weight" problem. Ironically, many are often uncomfortable when they receive approval for having lost weight, so they really are stuck between a rock and a hard place. They crave attention, but recoil from it when it's for shedding pounds or for carrying more weight than they'd like. What a dilemma!

• *Without an eating problem, carrying excess weight, or exhibiting poor self-care, how will people know that I'm a person of substance and not invisible?*

The issue of visibility versus invisibility comes up a good deal in my practice. Many disregulated eaters are conflicted about whether or not they want to be seen. If they were heavy as children, being seen may have meant being criticized. If they were teased about their weight, they might feel equally that being a large size makes them too visible and, therefore, a target for harassment.

Many disregulated eaters grew up in homes in which the best way to survive was to fly under their parents' radar whenever possible, that is, to make themselves invisible. At the first whiff of an argument between Mom and Dad, they'd dash up the stairs to their rooms (with a pint of ice cream in tow) or grab their coats and quietly sneak out of the house to visit a neighbor or sit on the stoop by themselves. Being invisible became a goal—a survival tool—but along with their unnoticed bodies went their unnoticed emotional needs. So being invisible became both a plus and a minus.

Along with the visibility versus invisibility dilemma comes one of power versus helplessness. If you're big and have substance and heft, you're less likely to be pushed around physically. However, this same bulk makes you stand out and feel powerless as a target for meanness. Although weight may say, "Look at me, I'm important, you can't mess with me," internally you want to disappear because you don't *feel* powerful at all. It's natural to desire to feel empowered, but that is best done through words and actions, not appearance.

Food for Thought

How do you feel about receiving positive attention? If it makes you uncomfortable, why is that? Growing up in your family, did you feel invisible or too visible—or a little of both?

• *Without an eating problem, carrying excess weight, or exhibiting poor self-care, how will people know that I'm struggling and trying to better myself?*

The majority of disregulated eaters engage in perpetual struggle. Their identities revolve around excelling and achieving. Not feeling good enough through simply being, they push themselves to *do* in order to raise their self-esteem.

If you were brought up to believe that you must work hard to succeed, you recognize that effort pays off. However, if you were raised to believe that you always must struggle to reach success and happiness, you're in a world of trouble. This kind of thinking leads you to believe that struggle is a goal in itself, and that if you feel satisfied and content, there's something wrong with you. People with a struggler identity hardly ever take the easy way out—I know, I used to be one of them. Obviously, we are all a work in progress; however, we need not be a struggle in progress.

If you're continuously losing and regaining weight, you may be conflicted about whether it's okay to not struggle over it. Giving up the battle may seem like a cop out. In that case, you may be stuck in a dilemma that goes like this: *It's a good thing that I'm always struggling to get my weight down and I'm a quitter if I don't keep fighting the good fight,* versus *I'm tired of struggling with my eating and my body and just want to make peace with my weight.*

I had a client in one of my eating workshops decades ago who had just received her Ph.D. and was honored with a significant monetary prize for some complicated research she'd spent most of her time doing. After graduation, her research complete (and the check for her prize money deposited in the bank), she was left with nothing to work on. She'd lost some weight during six of our eight weeks of class, but noticed that she was gradually putting it back on.

In class one night, she realized that she hated and was uneasy being without a goal. She then wondered if she might have (unconsciously) begun to gain weight to give herself another goal to work toward. The idea seemed strange to her, but made sense in terms of her upbringing and belief system. She talked in class about how, growing up, her overachieving parents had relentlessly pushed her to bust her butt to always be working on *something* or she would be considered lazy and unmotivated. She recalled how appalled they'd be even now if she gave up her struggle with food and her body and made peace with both.

By the end of the workshop, she decided that she wanted to try to experience life without major goals, including getting her body to a specific weight. She recognized that the uneasiness she currently felt being without goals was not a state to be avoided, but a learning experience, and wisely decided to see what it had to teach her.

Food for Thought

Were you brought up that pursuing goals is an absolute necessity? What would happen if you gave up struggling with weight? With eating? What might you learn from not pushing toward goals and relaxing a bit more into life?

• *Without an eating problem, carrying excess weight, or exhibiting poor self-care, how will people know that I want to be loved as is, as my perfectly imperfect self?*

Many disregulated eaters were raised in homes in which love was offered on a contingency basis only—I'll be proud of you *if* you get a top grade, lose weight, excel in sports, or become as perfect as you can be. The message from these parents is that if you do these things, then—*and only then*—will you deserve and receive love. My heart hurts writing about how common this dynamic is and for the damage it wreaks on budding egos, because when disregulated eaters don't receive unconditional love in childhood, they don't know how to give it to themselves in adulthood. Instead, they lack self-compassion and beat themselves up unmercifully.

I have an old friend, an eating disorder therapist, as it happens, who grew up with a mother who was extremely critical of her. If you had a parent who was controlling, domineering and judgmental, you know how unlovable this makes you feel as a child and how this perception carries right on into your adult years. In therapy, one day, this friend had an epiphany about her weight, which had crept up over the decades until it had become a health problem.

Although she had a prestigious job, loving family, and many friends, she realized that more than anything else she wanted people to love her as is. This meant she wished them to not want her to lose weight or care if she did, to see her as fine just as she was. I say this was an epiphany because it points up the conflict she'd had for decades: *I want to be loved as I am, at a size which is generally unacceptable to society and maybe even to myself, but if I lose weight, how will this ever happen?* Said another way, she believed she had to hold onto her weight or give up her quest for unconditional love.

• *Without an eating problem, carrying excess weight, or exhibiting poor self-care, if people still reject or abandon me, won't that mean I'm defective and there's something really wrong with me?*

The conflict generated by this question is quite common among disregulated eaters, many of whom feel defective in some way to begin with, eating and weight aside. Of course, most of them are unaware that they've always functioned on the assumption that something is wrong with them. If you come at life from this angle, weight becomes a very convenient target and shield. It's a target because if you don't receive a call back on a job interview or get asked out on a second date, you can *always* blame your weight. It's a shield because you don't have to dig below the surface to those rock-bottom, scary fears about how defective you *really* might be.

Please, please don't think I'm saying there *is* something defective about you. Not at all, that is, no more so than with everyone else on the planet. We're all imperfect. Those of us who know and accept this fact, and love ourselves dearly and deeply in spite of it, just take our inadequacies in stride. But folks who believe that they should be perfect and are ashamed of their imperfection are in a pickle. They can't reflect on their shortcomings and challenges without coming face to face with their worst fear: that their defects are unfixable.

This darker assumption often underlies mixed feelings about weight loss: *If I lose weight, I'll feel better about myself, but what if my size isn't causing my unhappiness and I have more deep-seated, unfixable deficits that people will see?* When you're choosing between a *known* enemy (perceived or real excess weight) versus an *unknown* one (an unfixable, intolerable self), you're facing a tough conflict to resolve.

Food for Thought

Do you blame your weight for your unhappiness? What else could make you unhappy if you were satisfied with your weight? Did you feel defective before you had eating or "weight" problems?

If I resolve my conflicted feelings about my identity, will I eat more "normally," lose weight, and take consistently good care of myself?

Resolving your conflicts is an excellent place to start moving toward taking better care of yourself, but there are a few more issues for you to clear up as well. Changing your identity isn't like turning on a light switch or charging out of a phone booth like Clark Kent turning into Superman. Would that it were so easy. There are several issues, perhaps more accurately called fears, that might get in the way of transforming who you are (and who you think you are) into who you want to be. Exploring them will help you clarify your beliefs and point you in a direction to alter them if need be. As I said in earlier chapters, many of our fears lurk outside of our awareness. Acknowledging that you hold some of these fears is the first step in overcoming them.

• *What if people still don't love me if I'm thinner?*

Well, what if they don't? I assure you that, as you go through life, there will be some people who can take or leave you, and a handful who may actively dislike you. That's life, and it won't matter very much in the long run because most people will probably like you and a few will love you dearly, and you'll gravitate to them (at least I *hope* you will!). Keep in mind that there are men and women out there who will dislike you because of your job, politics, religion, and education (or lack thereof), and other individuals who will like or love you for exactly these same reasons!

For example, I can sometimes be outspoken and there are people who value this trait in me and others who don't. Also, I try to see both sides of an issue, which one friend calls being wishy-washy, but others think shows open minded-ness. The truth is, even serial killers might be liked by some people. Honestly, what could be so bad about you that people would get to know you and turn away? If you greatly fear people not liking what they see when you become more intimate, could your problem be an underlying, mistaken feeling of defectiveness (which was covered in chapter six)?

I had a client decades ago who was a handsome, high energy man who was repeatedly told by women that he was "too intense." Years after we ended therapy, I received an email from him saying that he'd moved to Canada and found a wonderful woman who loved him precisely because he was so passionate about life! No matter what your size, weight, or personality—no matter how well you take care of yourself—there are bound to be folks who simply don't take a shine to you and people who do.

Do you like every thin person you meet? C'mon. Cut yourself some slack and don't make it all about you—especially your weight. Put your best foot forward and see what happens. As I said before, weight discrimination is rampant in America. I'm not trying to sugar-coat this fact for you, especially if you are large. But there are plenty of big people in great relationships and great jobs and plenty of thin or average-sized folks in terrible jobs and awful relationships. Ultimately, size has little to do with personal fulfillment or happiness.

• *What if people are jealous of me when I'm thinner and take good care of myself?*

I can't tell you there won't be folks who'll resent that you're healthier than they are. I can give you two personal examples. Example one. When I lost about 20 pounds through "normal" eating gradually in the course of my thirties, I recall being at a party in Beacon Hill, a tony part of Boston. I was self-conscious about my thinner body and agonized about what to wear: Should I throw on something that covered up my shape or get all dolled up and let my body look like, well, my body? I went for the latter.

On the buffet line, a man and I started chatting, just making small talk about our hostess or some inconsequential topic. After we'd gotten our food, we went our separate ways. Later that night, the hostess told me that this man's wife had pulled her aside and complained, "What was that 'thin' woman doing talking to my husband?" I felt badly, but knew I'd done nothing untoward and didn't feel responsible for this wife's insecurities ostensibly caused by my "thinness."

Example two. Later in life, I joined a women's group and was meeting people for the first time. At the start of the meeting, I did the usual bit of rising and introducing myself. I mentioned my move from Boston and being a psychotherapist and the author of books on eating and weight and left it at that. After the meeting, a bunch of women went out for drinks and not a one asked me to join them. I tagged along anyway.

A few days later, I asked a friend, a member of the group who hadn't been there that night, about the cold-shoulder I'd received. Her take was that maybe some of the women didn't like the fact that I was on the thin side or were envious that I was a published author (several of them were in the writing field). Since then, I'm glad to say that I've become friends with many of these women and who weighs what or has written what hasn't been an issue for any of us.

None of us can control how people feel about us. Also, their reactions may change over time. Haven't you ever been turned off at first meeting someone and down the road grown to like them? Or vice versa? So, yes, people might dislike you because you're working on becoming healthier—and look it. But it's more likely that people who take good care of themselves will be drawn to you precisely because of your positive self-care behaviors. Think about it: Would you not pursue lofty educational or high-paying occupations because folks might think you're arrogant or materialistic? I hope not.

• *What if I lose weight, spruce up my appearance, and become like the stereotype of thin people—cold, snooty, and selfish—even though I'm not really like that?*

This is a common fear of disregulated eaters, that they'll not only lose the traits they love about themselves if they focus more on taking care of themselves, but that their bodies will somehow be taken over by an alien thin persona. Do you know many people who've changed in this way? Have you lost weight and done a personality switch-er-oo yourself? Remember, stereotypes abound around weight, skin color, ethnicity, geographic region, and religion. Changing your outsides doesn't mean changing your insides.

One of the reasons that weight loss and ongoing self-care won't turn you into someone you don't want to be is exactly that: you don't want to be that way. Most people, no matter what their weight is who are cold, snooty, and selfish probably either don't recognize this fact or don't care. You, however, will work diligently not to think or act in ways that are counter to your values. Please stop worrying about being taken over by pod people.

Perhaps your fears are more about what *you* think about fat and thin than what other people do. Now is the time to acknowledge and come to terms with your own fat phobia—

not tomorrow or if your weight changes. Either you hate fat bodies, yours included, or you don't, have compassion for people with weight struggles or contempt, value all shapes and sizes or use them to negatively evaluate people. This is why eating disorder experts encourage us to value size diversity and accept our bodies as they are—because fat prejudice and over-valuing thinness is a barrier to becoming a mentally healthy person no matter what our weight.

Meet Louise and Her Conflict

The facts:

The first thing I noticed about Louise was her wise-cracking, maybe because I occasionally enjoy being a smart-mouth myself. During our first session, among other things, she joked about the difference in our size—I'm petite and she weighed over 300 pounds. She'd never been in therapy before, she reported, and rattled off some basic facts about herself before I had a chance to ask: "I'm 59, I grew up in Brooklyn, I'm fat, my whole family's fat, I'm a bookkeeper at (she named an upscale restaurant in Boston), I own my own condo, I was widowed in my early 30s, and I have one daughter who's gay and lives in New Hampshire with her partner."

When I asked how I could help her, Louise joked that she wanted to take off a few pounds. I took an eating/weight history as I always do, and Louise said her entire family is, was, and as far as she could tell, would always be obsessed with food. As a child, her father had owned a deli in Brooklyn and brought home the most luscious delicacies every night—knishes, strudel, white fish, and rugelach. She and her siblings would wait for him to close the store and come home, which meant eating late. She said that sometimes, out of hunger, she snacked until he arrived, but ate whatever he brought home anyway; other times she rode out her hunger (he sometimes came home as late as eight o'clock) but practically fell on the food when her father set it out on the table.

She described her parents, maternal and paternal grandparents, and two brothers as large. Most of her cousins were big like her, except for a few "skinny" cousins whom, she swore, no one liked. When I raised the issue of having a family identity, she said that, without a doubt, theirs was food based. When they went on vacation, at breakfast, they'd discuss where they'd go to lunch, then at lunch, they'd talk about which restaurant to try for dinner.

Louise said that in her twenties, she'd made her one and only foray into the diet world when she met her husband who, oddly enough, she added, was thin as a rail. She said for the first time in her life, she wanted to be thin, or at least thin*ner* and succeeded for about two years minding her weight, until her husband was diagnosed with bone cancer and died. She said she might have been able to continue to watch what she ate except that, with a job and young daughter, she decided to move back to her parents' home and "my weight became a lost cause."

I asked about her current bookkeeping job at a local restaurant and she sighed and said that her office was above it on the second floor, and that she ate almost all her meals downstairs. She felt blessed with delicious food, all for free, and admitted that she ate without discretion, finding it mildly amusing that "all my life, I can't get away from food."

Louise's conflict:

It's easy to see how Louise's entire identity revolved around food and eating from her childhood right through adulthood. In photos, it was obvious that everyone in the family was hefty and she didn't recall that her parents or brothers ever had tried to lose weight, at least that she knew of. As we talked about how her identity was wrapped around food, Louise became sad, feeling hopeless that she could ever change. She admitted that she couldn't imagine not having food as the center of her world or feeling comfortable at a lower weight. Her weight symbolized her whole life and she was afraid of losing a major part of her identity if she looked in the mirror and her reflection didn't fill up most of the glass.

She worried that even if she did manage to take off weight she would no longer fit in with her family. Unable to visualize attending a holiday dinner and not eating all the scrumptious dishes and divine desserts, she finally broke down and started to cry. Talk about conflicts, it was painful to see how torn Louise was. She suddenly realized that worry about not fitting in with her family was one of the main factors preventing her from regulating her eating. She saw clearly how her mixed feelings had been a barrier all along and decided to at least try to resolve them.

The resolution:

I knew that Louise needed support if she was going to make headway with "normal" eating and she was willing to try almost anything I suggested. First, I got her hooked up with a registered dietician who could help her focus on adding nutritious foods to her diet. Between them, they decided that Louise would eat only one meal a day at the restaurant, whichever she chose, but only one. Her other two meals would be eaten at home and planned out ahead of time.

Louise also agreed to go to a support group to learn "normal" eating, which gave her a new identity: a potential "normal" eater. We both agreed that having her involved with people who were attempting to eat differently and become healthier was a necessity if she were to create an identity other than "overeater" or "fat person" for herself. This group also was intended to be a counter-weight (pardon the pun) to her family.

Louise enjoyed the group so much that she went with some of the members to a few weekend retreats which focused on mindful eating. To my surprise, this bubbly, outgoing woman totally enjoyed the silent, meditative meals at some of the retreats. This was the first time in her life she said that she'd paid any attention to the process of eating. It was a whole new world for her. When she finally felt ready, Louise went home to visit her parents for the holidays. Terrified doesn't begin to describe how she felt. We arranged for her to keep a journal during the visit, and that I would be on call if she wanted to talk to me.

To her great surprise, her relatives noticed her weight loss of about 30 pounds ("Would you believe they told me my face looked too thin!") and listened as she explained that she was trying to lose weight for her health. She also made a point of asking them not to comment on her eating which some were able to do and some weren't. She said she felt as loved and as much a part of the family as she always had, and that she didn't eat perfectly but she ate far better than she ever dreamed she could around them. Over time, as Louise began to eat more "normally," she acknowledged missing her old ways of eating because they'd been such a significant part of her life, but also found tremendous satisfaction in being able to make such a major, positive shift in her identity.

HOMEWORK

Write out these answers for yourself.

1. What did you learn about your conflicts with your identity?

2. What ideas and concepts were new to you?

3. Which made you feel better or more hopeful?

4. Which made you feel uncomfortable or anxious?

5. What specific actions can you take to feel more comfortable with who you are, how you see yourself, and the image you project?

MOVING FORWARD

CHAPTER ELEVEN

RESOLVE INTERNAL CONFLICTS FOR GOOD

(I'm Gonna Sit Here and Break Bread with Myself!)

By now, I hope you understand that achieving a permanent, positive relationship with food relies upon resolving your internal conflicts. This chapter provides you with a bag of take-along tools for your journey that will support your resolve and provide you with the resources needed to reach your goals. Remember, this book is about creating lasting change from the inside out, which means restructuring your inner world—your thoughts and feelings—to reboot your brain and retrain behavior.

My hunch is that many of you tried to speed read through this book to quickly "get" what I have to say, though you know that impatience is a major impediment to recovery. Your habit has been to dive into fixing whatever isn't working rather than allow time for the process of change to take its course. If you're still fixated on *being* there rather than *getting* there, you might benefit from going back to the seven keys, reading through them again, and really taking time to digest my words and answer the questions at the end of every section—actually write out your homework answers at the end of each key chapter. Remember, pushing yourself to speed through this book or your recovery will actually slow the process down.

Now that you understand that internal conflicts have been holding you back and that there's a path to resolving them, my guess is that you still require a bit more assistance in getting the job done. Well, here goes. You know how when you're planning a trip—trekking cross country or traveling abroad—you must first think about what you need for your journey and who might accompany you? This chapter provides you with a laundry list of the *internal companions* you'll want to take along.

You'll want the following personality traits with you every step of the way. If you don't have them, you'll need to develop them, but it's worth it, because they're all necessary and will lead to improving your quality of life.

• Mindful curiosity

If you can come at this work with genuine curiosity about your polarized thinking, you won't waste time with self-judgment when you bump into facets of yourself you're not too wild about. Curiosity means wanting both to scour the hidden nooks and crannies of your psyche for enlightening discoveries, and to respond with neutrality to whatever you find. I'm sure there are aspects of life you're curious about—travel, science, history, literature, or political science—in which you feel no need to pronounce judgment every time you come across new bits of information.

Well, that's the attitude to have. If you're pleased with your discoveries as you learn about what makes you tick, terrific; and if you're not pleased, still terrific, because every new bit of data is useful in deciphering what's going on in your mind and heart. Any time self-judgment arises, just shrug it off and set your curiosity cap back squarely on your head. Curiosity drives insight and none of us can have too much of that! Remember that awareness may come as an ah-ha moment or sneak up on you gradually.

Too many people sleep-race through life, rushing from this task to that, ticking perceived demands off their to-do list as if their lives depended on it, and forgetting that the only time that is ever ours is the present. As you learn about yourself, make sure to remain connected to the here and now. When your mind tries to leap ahead, desperate to know all the answers before it possibly can, lasso it back and calm it down. Remember that the past and future are mental constructs while now is reality.

• Reflection and insight

Which kind of people are more mentally healthy: those who are self-reflective or those who aren't? You don't need a degree in psychology to answer that question correctly. Self-reflection is one the most effective tools humans can employ to solve their problems. For example, I ran into a gentleman recently who'd started a business and realized too late that he didn't have the skills required to make it a success. He had a fine product, but hated marketing and couldn't give a sales pitch to save his life. Moreover, he lacked the funds to hire someone to do what he couldn't or wouldn't do. Had he spent time reflecting on the type of person he was rather than charging full steam ahead with his product idea hoping he'd change, he wouldn't have invested thousands of dollars and months of time in production of his prototype. Self-reflection would have saved him a wad of money, a lot of grief, and a heap of disappointment.

Studies show that reflective people have a tick that may indicate they're thinking deeply: When asked a question that requires consideration, they automatically roll their eyes upward before answering, as if they're trying to turn inward to "see" a worthwhile response. Isn't this exactly how we draw a cartoon character deep in thought?

Ask yourself: Am I reflective? Here are some questions to help you decide. Do you consider all possible consequences before taking action? Do you spend time wondering (not judging!) how you feel or what you think about a subject before responding to an important question? Do you look to your own intuition to seek solutions within rather than rush off to solicit others' opinions? Do you use both your thoughts and feelings as you maneuver through life? Self-reflection is a habit which is essential for everyone, and is especially necessary for disregulated eaters who tend to look for quick fixes outside themselves.

Insight, which comes from reflection, is a deep understanding of self and others. It helps you synthesize information to gain clarity about how your past has affected your present and how your present might affect your future. Although people can be taught to develop insight, many folks seem to come by it naturally and it's an asset like none other. If you think of yourself as an insightful person, great; if not, work on developing this facility as you continue to address your food problems.

But, please remember, insight is not all that is necessary for recovery. Too many people make brilliant connections and observations and have amazing epiphanies about why they eat as they do, but don't do anything transformative with the information. Insight is what starts the game of change, and practicing new ways of thinking and behaving is what carries you over the finish line.

• Self-honesty

To achieve your goals, it's crucial to look at yourself squarely and say, "I don't like what I see, but that's me, all right!" Naturally, it's more difficult to look at aspects of ourselves that we dislike than those we like, but nothing is more important for teasing out ambivalence than embracing our fears and inadequacies.

We bury aspects of self that we're uncomfortable with and try to keep them buried because they make us uncomfortable. If you think of yourself as a victim and hate that about yourself, all right, bring that aspect of self into the light and have a good look-see at what's behind it. Learning about the "worst" in you is bound to bring out the best!

• Self-compassion

The one major trait that practically all disregulated eaters sorely lack is self-compassion. In my 30 some years of working with troubled eaters, I've never met one who didn't exude its opposite, self-judgment or, worse, self-contempt. Their hearts go out to others, but they are positively merciless toward themselves. The good news is that empathy toward others indicates that you understand and value caring. The bad news is that you probably don't feel worthy of applying it toward yourself.

Occasionally, I do run into troubled eaters who lack compassion, period. They pretty much feel contempt for anyone (themselves included) who doesn't live up to their standards—and what impossibly high standards they are. These folks need to work on allowing themselves to feel caring in spite of imperfection and let their compassion, which is a natural feeling, replace contempt, which is a learned one.

So many of you show yourselves no mercy, especially in the eating and weight arena and that's one of the reasons you're stuck. You hate your: body, lack of control, failures, and obsession with food. You're terrified that if you show compassion to yourself for your inadequacies, you won't change, but you've failed to notice that all the contempt you've thrown at yourself hasn't exactly brought you the success you so desperately desire.

Paradoxically, the key to resolving your mixed feelings is to embrace the traits in yourself that have prevented you from reaching your goals. That means *always* showering yourself with self-compassion.

You need not like or agree with every one of your thoughts and feelings. You don't have to go out and celebrate that you're easily frustrated and have difficulty delaying gratification, or that you're virtually clueless about how to comfort yourself without food. Just bring your awareness to the truths of who you are, and know that you're working to change them. Recognize that you're allowed to be flawed.

I spent the first third of my life lacking self-compassion and I've tried my best to live out the rest of it practicing it every minute of every day. I even have compassion for the times I don't show myself compassion! The compassion you feel toward your least favorite traits is the prime catalyst for changing them.

• Willingness to learn by experience

Another trait often missing in disregulated eaters is a willingness to learn from experience. In part, this is because you're so busy beating yourselves up for what you perceive as your mistakes. This is why curiosity, honesty, and compassion are crucial. The first question to ask yourself after you eat half an apple pie isn't, "How can I be such a jerk?" but, "What was going on with me that I disrespected my appetite and hurt myself?" You learn to value your experience by taking the time to examine and make sense of it. Remember, judgment has no place in this process.

Here are examples of learning by experience. Say you didn't get your teeth cleaned on schedule and consequently have a bunch of cavities. By recognizing that avoiding the dentist was a poor decision, you can now set an intention to make and keep more appointments in the future. Or maybe you stopped your weekend golf game and daily walks and now huff and puff when you walk up the stairs. You've learned something: it's time to resume your activities. You can never go wrong with asking yourself why something happened. If nothing else, examination feels a lot better than flagellation.

One other point about learning from experience: Be careful about casting your past in concrete. Use the skill of self-reflection to figure out what you could have done better *last* time and what you could improve *next* time. Consider new problem solving-strategies, then monitor them and evaluate how they're working. Be flexible and try any reasonable, healthy approach that will help resolve your internal conflicts. Avoid saying, "See, my history is a string of failures, so why try again?" Things change, we change.

Reflect, be honest, take action, assess, and learn from experience without judging it.

• Patience

How are you going to get the best answers for yourself if you rush the discovery process? Better to slow down. Patience helps you tolerate the trial-and-error nature of change—this didn't work, but okay, maybe that will. Impatience is one of *the* major barriers to succeeding at "normal" eating. Haven't you noticed that the more you yearn for "recovery," the slower it happens? You are going as fast as you can!

I recently heard an interview with a multi-media artist who clearly had his head on straight. The interviewer asked him how he knew in advance the length of time a project would take. His answer was that he never knew, and that his only interest was putting out a work that was the best he could do whether it took "two weeks, two months or two years." Clone that attitude for yourself!

I know you want to feel better about your self-care abilities, but changing your view of yourself to worthwhile and perfectly imperfect does not happen overnight. I wish I *could* make it happen with a snap of my fingers, but that's not how life works. Nor can you awaken one morning and totally change your identity (that only happens in the movies). None of the conflicts in this book is going to resolve in a matter of days or weeks.

When you're trying to figure out if you've eaten enough, patience will help you determine your body's fullness and whether you feel satisfied. Then you'll need more patience to check in and notice how your body feels right after eating, two hours later, and several hours after that. Getting to know yourself and other people takes time, so try not to be impulsive or force decisions before you're ready to make them. You'll get there when you get there.

• Persistence and practice

Nearing the end of this book, you may be wondering if you have the stick-to-itiveness to reach your eating, weight, and self-care goals. You'll have to be curious and engage in honest self-reflection to come up with your answer. Remember, identifying your mixed feelings is only the *beginning* of the process.

Persistence gently prods you forward even when you feel as if you're not making progress. It's another name for exhibiting faith in your worthy self. When you're persistent, practicing new attitudes and behaviors becomes easier over time. Practice is what takes you *from* understanding your conflicting feelings about, say, giving up food for comfort *to* establishing new ways to manage stress and distress. Practice comes more easily when you have some or all of the previously mentioned traits. For example, curiosity, self-honesty, and insight help you identify barriers to moving forward. Patience and self-compassion make it possible to applaud yourself for each baby step you make in the right direction.

• Trusting others and asking for help

Last but not least, you will be well served by learning to trust others and ask for help when you need it. There is no set way of knowing whether to sit with a problem and try to figure it out on your own or seek outside counsel. Self is *always* the place to start, but it's fine if you end up going to others for suggestions or feedback. What you don't want to do is either ask them before you've tried to sort things out on your own or never ask them because you don't want to look stupid or bother someone.

Here's an example of how the process might go. I was struggling with an ethical dilemma regarding having a family member of an ex-client come to see me. I tossed the issue back and forth debating if I would be violating clinical boundaries and causing myself problems down the line. Unable to make up my mind, I emailed several therapist friends and laid out the dilemma. Rather than being ashamed to show them my indecisiveness, I was thrilled to have trusted colleagues to whom I could go for advice.

Discussing any of your conflicts with even one person would be a great start. Other people can give us a perspective that we simply cannot have on our own. I can't tell you how often someone will offer some bit of wisdom and I think how wonderful it is that we can all help each other. I'm so often reminded how narrow my view of the world is and am grateful that everyone doesn't see life as I do. As the saying goes, we can't see the picture when we're inside the frame.

Food for Thought

Which of the above traits come naturally to you, and which ones do you need to work on? Please take time to look at each trait separately, with curiosity and without judgment about what you discover. You can improve in all these skill areas.

Is there anything I can do to speed up the change process just a teensy bit?

There is one more thing to learn about and it's called the *organic process*. Many people have no idea what this is, and if you think it's something having to do with farming, you're not far off. The term *organic process* most often describes biological occurrences involving absorption, growth, adaptation, synthesis, maturation, and metamorphosis, words that evoke a sense of change that seems natural, gradual, and almost inevitable. Using the organic process, you follow your major and minor leanings—thoughts and feelings—however and wherever they roam, until through synthesis, they naturally coalesce to an acceptable outcome.

Although the organic process is most often used to describe how changes occur in our physical world, it's spot on in describing the path to psychological transformation as well. Key elements of this method include:

- natural progression rather than decisions through urgency or predetermination

- every action arising as an outgrowth of the previous action or actions

- a sense of natural order and logic

- assessments based on neutrality rather than values of "good" or "bad"

- unfolding, rather than forced, movement or progression that includes narrowing down options from the general to the specific

Here's an example of how to use the organic process. Let's say you're thinking about where to move your family. You'd first consider where you can get a job and where housing would suit your needs. After that, you might look at what geographic areas have the elements you're looking for in terms of quality of life—climate, transportation, clean air, schools, and safety. Finally, you'd whittle down your choices to a few cities or towns. See the flow from general to specific. Notice that there's no urgency to come to a "right" decision, no need to force a choice, to have all the details nailed down before you come to an end point—no need even to know where you're going until you mentally get there. This gradual discovery or unfolding is a hallmark of the organic process.

The key to using the organic process to resolve internal conflicts is not having a stake in the outcome other than resolution, a difficult process for disregulated eaters, who tend to be highly goal-oriented with a fear of doing the wrong thing. For instance, you don't have to know exactly how you'll stop feeling defective and start feeling deserving; instead, simply start moving in that direction and see what comes of it. Using the "where should I move my family analogy" at the start of the process, you don't need to know *where* you'll be moving, only that you will assuredly find someplace suitable.

The how happens as you follow the natural progression of your thoughts, feelings, and actions. As you reflect, you get jazzed up by some ideas and turned off by others. Some that started on the top of the heap, sink to the bottom while others which seemed insignificant bubble their way upward. Still other ideas keep on circling around and you find you are unable to let them go. In the organic process, one thing leads to another. Using the moving-your-family example, let's say that as you're cleaning the attic, you come across a photo of a vacation spot you loved when you were six. You remember having dreams of the quaint mountain town where you stayed, somewhere with a waterfall nearby, and this image gets you thinking about how much you want to live near water. In fact, that thought jumps out at you, clear as day, and you wonder how you didn't realize long ago how crucial being by a body of water is to you. You don't minimize this desire or idea as unrealistic; instead, you take it seriously because it resonates deeply within you.

The organic process is the equivalent of *mindful living.* You stay acutely tuned in to all your senses and gut feelings, check out everything initially, lead with curiosity and avoid making anything right or wrong, listen to what others have to say but have confidence that you know what's best for yourself. You don't try to push the river; rather you willingly, joyfully flow along with it.

More than any other factors, the organic process requires curiosity and patience. Curiosity is necessary to rid yourself of shoulds and judgments that pull you away from authentic desire. Patience is essential because you will not get an instant answer. Think evolution, not revolution. Here's the trade-off: Your answer won't be quick, but it will be just right for you.

You may have difficulty engaging in the organic process, because it requires tolerance of ambiguity and uncertainty—not knowing how or when you'll arrive at a satisfactory outcome. You'll have to give up interest in having "the right answer" and knowing how things will turn out. Think of the organic process as following a trail of breadcrumbs made up of your thoughts and feelings—even your dreams. What's best for you will eventually make itself known and, paradoxically, will feel like an answer that has been part of you all along.

Food for Thought

Explain the organic process as you understand it. What are its key elements? How does it differ from the way you make decisions now?

Here are specific steps to resolving your conflicts:

Step #1: Observe without judgment

Be an observer of your own thoughts and behavior. Look for alerts that something is going on within you. No need to work yourself up into a lather. Just put on your curiosity cap and say, "Well, now, isn't it interesting that I tell myself *not* to take that left which brings me to the fast food drive-through every day on the way home from work and, yet, here I am like clockwork."

Step #2: Identify your conflict

After you've identified that you have a conflict occurring, dig around a little so you can understand it. You might say, "I get it. On the one hand, after work, I'm too tired to start preparing dinner, so I get fast food because it's easy and quick." *However,* "I also want to be healthy and the foods I eat there make me feel bloated and not very satisfied later in the evening. Plus I could kick myself for eating junk." There you have it, your dilemma isn't so much about food as about better managing stress and the transition from home to work. Your conflict is based on ambivalence about how best to take care of yourself.

Step #3: Anticipate your conflict

Simply recognizing that you have polarized feelings and identifying what they are won't cut it in the do-things-differently department. To change, you want to remain vigilant. Therefore, you might awaken in the morning and remind yourself that you're going to be exhausted after work and will likely head for the drive-thru unless you have a healthier plan when you leave the office. You might then dig out something from the freezer for dinner before leaving home or make time at lunch to buy some healthy groceries. It would also help to stop during the day and visualize arriving home and enjoying the healthy meal you've planned.

Step #4: Watch your language

The language I'm talking about here are your old friends: should, have to, need to, ought to, must, and supposed to. Drop them like a hot potato. Instead, replace them with: want, would like, wish, desire, or prefer. Don't say, "I *should* go home and make myself that nice piece of tilapia I took out of the freezer this morning." Say, "I want to go to the drive-through, and I also want to go home and eat the tilapia." Notice how these are both internal desires. Well, fair enough, may the best decision win. If some external words sneak into your self-talk, just repeat your wish with internal words, and you're good to go.

Step #5: Do yourself proud

Whenever there's a decision to be made, ask yourself, "Will doing this make me proud or ashamed in the long run?" Don't worry about the content of the choice or over-analyze your options. The issue is how you're going to feel about doing something one way or the other. So, as you leave work, be thinking about how you'll feel if you stop for fast food versus patiently waiting for the tilapia. Once you remove the should-shouldn't debate, with all its intense emotional baggage, you are in a position to make a choice between two desires, and choose the one that would make you proud.

Step #6: Keep patting yourself on the back

After you make a healthy decision and any time after that, marinate yourself in pride. Give yourself three cheers! Do not ignore your triumph. Accentuate the positive, even if it feels uncomfortable to dwell on doing well. Don't tell yourself your choice was no big deal, you should have done it anyway. Be proud and stay proud! Remember, nothing tastes as good as pride.

At some point, if you continue to put effort into getting to know yourself inside and out, your major conflicts about eating, weight, and self-care will resolve. And if new conflicts pop up, you'll know just what to do to identify and dispense with them. Of course, you'll still have the usual ups and downs that make life interesting and keep you on your toes, but you'll approach new challenges with clarity about your self-worth and confidence that you know how to take care of yourself. You'll whole-heartedly want to eat according to the rules of "normal" eating and insist on the absolute best for your body. You'll treat your entire being from head to toe with nothing but respect and loving care. This will be your new identity, your way of life, automatic and tremendously satisfying.

That's the gift of hard work and self-discovery!

CHAPTER TWELVE

FURTHER
SELF-DISCOVERY

(I'm Getting Smarter by the Minute!)

I want you to think of finishing this book as the beginning of a new approach to eating and self-care. Now that you've identified your internal conflicts, the words "Starting Monday" take on a whole different meaning, one that promises real and permanent change.

To speed you along, this chapter contains a slew of ideas to ponder and activities to try, as you move toward attaining and maintaining your health and fitness goals.

KEY #1

Create Lasting Change

• Reframe your irrational beliefs about change to rational ones using the first person and the present tense. Do this with at least a half dozen beliefs. Read them aloud often, and add more as you discover them.

• Put up a big sign in your brain that says, "Baby steps, baby steps, baby steps."

• Stop saying, "This is hard," or "I can't do this," about changing your self-care habits. This only programs your brain to think that change is difficult. Reprogram by saying, "This is challenging but doable," "I can do this with a little more effort," or "I'll get there."

• Consider how your parents modeled change when you were growing up. Notice if they insisted that you be patient but didn't practice what they preached, which is confusing for a child. If your parents are alive, observe how they deal with change now.

• Use a timeline to outline in detail one or two ways you've changed in the past. Look at the stages you traveled through to end up with new attitudes and behaviors, paying special attention to the times when you reverted to old habits, and how you renewed your motivation to finally reach your goals.

• Make a list of the traits you believe will facilitate realistic change (such as the ones in the beginning of this chapter) and decide how to go about acquiring each one.

• Be more curious than judgmental. Rather than having a strong, good or bad opinion on what you see and hear in life, stay neutral and wonder about what's happening. Cheer every step you take toward your goals and minimize your mistakes and failures.

• To keep yourself present and aware, stay grounded in your body as much as possible by focusing on your senses. Check in frequently about what you see, hear, smell, taste, and feel through touch and what emotions you're feeling. Be aware of when you put pressure on yourself to change more quickly than is possible, and use self-talk to slow yourself down and take the pressure off.

• You can increase being reflective by not automatically responding to inquiries or demands. Instead, take a breath, tilt your eyes upward and inward and take a minute to pause.

• Put effort into being honest with yourself and not copping out. If you're wrong, admit it and be proud you did. Self-honesty need not hurt. Remind yourself that it helps in the long run.

• Practice self-compassion every minute of every day. Turn off the negative chatter about yourself that you'd never say to another soul—living or dead. Be as kind to, loving, comforting, and forgiving of yourself as you would be to a small child you loved—or to your dog or cat.

• You will always have opportunities to practice patience, so make sure your self-talk is soothing. Replace "I've got to finish this," with "It'll get done when I am ready and the time is right." Take deep breaths when you feel rushed and reduce inner pressure by reminding yourself you're only one human being doing your best.

• Notice when you want to give up and decide what you want to do about it. Sometimes the answer is to keep going and other times it's to stop because you've had enough for the time being. Cultivate persistence by acknowledging frustration, taking a break, reminding yourself of your goals, and being your own best cheerleader—all the while knowing you will continue moving forward at a later time.

• Practice is in a class by itself. Set a goal to do something X times a day or week. See how you make out. Make practice fun, like an adventure, not a tedious chore. Notice what stands in the way of practice—your thoughts or your environment—and change whatever needs to be changed.

• When you're stuck and you've exhausted your own inner resources, get help. If you're not used to seeking help, you may initially be uncomfortable. So what? This is a necessary life skill for everyone on the planet.

• Look for progress, not perfection. Mark progress by 1) increased frequency of healthy behavior, 2) decreased intensity of unhealthy behavior, 3) shorter periods of time engaging in unhealthy behavior. Aim for a balanced view, neither magnifying your tiniest shortcomings nor minimizing your biggest successes. Look for the things you're doing well!

• Work on extending your tolerance for frustration and delaying gratification. If you want a piece of candy now, make yourself wait 1 minute, then 5, then 10 and so on. You are an adult who can do this. Put your adult mind to work.

• Look at "mistakes" or "relapses" as learning opportunities and nothing else. After reflection, insight, or problem-solving, move on immediately.

KEY #2

Make Conscious Choices

• When you insist you have to do something, ask yourself why that is so, and "Who says?"

• Where in your body do you feel anger when you tell yourself you "must" do things? Notice if it's in your chest, neck, back, gut, or shoulders and relax that part of your body. Keep relaxing until you feel a release of tension.

• Replace the words should/must/ought to/need to/have to/am supposed to with desire/want/prefer/wish/would like to. Listen for how you talk to yourself and make sure you're always using internal motivators.

• When you want to fight what's best for you, ask yourself, "Who am I hurting?" Go look in the mirror and you'll see.

• Reframe your irrational beliefs about your ability to make choices to rational ones using the first person and the present tense. Move away from having a victim mentality. You're an adult and at least as big as your parents. This is one time to take off your baby shoes and put on your big girl or boy shoes.

• When you feel entitled to something that's unhealthy for you, stop and pay attention to the anger in the feeling. What or who are you angry at? When you've eaten the food or watched the TV programs, how long will you feel good about your decision? At whom will you be angry then?

• Make a list of healthy rewards for when you absolutely need one.

• Put up a set of photos or pictures of you fighting yourself and draw boxing gloves on your hands. Have a good laugh.

• When you're angry, don't take it out on yourself; you're allowed to be upset with others and confront them. You're less likely to turn your anger inward if you express it appropriately toward another person.

• Make a list of all the people who've tried to pressure, control and dominate you from childhood on. How would it help to let your anger go? Fantasize putting your anger into a balloon and letting it sail away. Being angry only hurts you, not them.

KEY #3

Feel Deserving

• Ask each of your friends to make a list of reasons you are deserving of the best in life and have them read it to you even if it makes you uncomfortable. Have them continue to read their list until you can hear it and feel comfortable. Save these lists and read them aloud for greater impact when you're having a bad day.

• Make a huge effort to take care of yourself even when you don't feel deserving (especially when you don't feel deserving), and pay attention to how much better you feel when you're proud of yourself.

• Write a paragraph or two about what makes a human being deserving and read it aloud to yourself. Keep it on hand for when you're feeling crummy.

• Make a list of unappealing traits in people you love, then decide which of these people are so defective they're undeserving or unlovable.

• Think back to your childhood to a time you didn't feel defective or undeserving. When exactly did this mistaken idea creep into your view of yourself? Make a list of your parents' unhealthy personality traits and another list of those belonging to your grandparents, aunts, and uncles. Do their faults make them undeserving or unlovable? What flaws are endearing?

• Rather than saying, "I deserve to eat this or that," remind yourself that of course you deserve to, but that's beside the point. Change, "I deserve to eat this" to "I can eat this if I am hungry and crave it."

• Have a debate with yourself or someone else about whether thin or fat people are more deserving of the good things in life. Back up your opinion with evidence and facts.

• Read books on loving yourself at any weight.

• Stop comparing yourself to what you perceive as others' "perfection." Come up with a phrase to remind yourself that everyone has flaws, like "Imperfect and proud of it!"

• Reflect on caring about something that isn't in good shape, like a sports team that's not doing well or an animal from a shelter. What makes imperfection tug at our hearts—and why aren't your imperfections tugging at yours?

• Make a list of all the non-material things you deserve in life and post it on your mirror or dashboard to read. This doesn't mean you're entitled to these things, just deserving of them.

• Every time you do something around food, weight, or self-care that disappoints you, give yourself a quick hug and big smile. This will help rewire your brain.

KEY #4

Comfort Yourself Effectively

• Count the times in a day you make statements that highlight your stress like, "I'm overwhelmed" or, "I've got to do this or that."

Put a penny in a jar for each time you misspeak and keep it handy!

• Make a list of your irrational beliefs about comforting yourself and coping with stress and distress—and reframe them.

• Be a student of behavior and observe the many ways people handle upset. Do they get angry, withdraw, blame or shame others, eat, drink, have a cigarette, take a nap, veg out in the front of the TV, take a walk? If you know them well, interview them about their methods: Did they always handle emotions well, how did they learn, do they have any tips for you?

• Which emotions give you the most trouble? Examine them one by one and explore what is so troublesome about any particular feeling. Be curious and don't judge yourself for not dealing well with it. If you'd had better teachers, you'd be more skilled. Good thing you're an adult now and can teach yourself.

• Read my *Food and Feelings Workbook* and do all the exercises in it!

• Make a list of situations and people that are triggering along with what you could do other than eat or engage in unhealthy activities.

• Other than eat, list 10 activities that comfort you.

• Identify the people in your life you can go to for comfort. Have three circles—an inner circle whom you'd trust with your life, a second that includes people you think would be able to help you feel better, and a third circle of people you could turn to if no one else was around.

• Write out a script of what you want to say to yourself the next time you're upset. Keep a few copies handy: in the kitchen, in your car, and on your cell phone or portable device.

• Make a list of five ways to reduce stress in each area of your life: family, work, community.

• Make a list of the ways you comfort others. Do you use these same strategies with yourself? If not, start now.

• Consider what's comforting about food—a distraction from emotions, momentary soothing, or a dopamine rush—and brainstorm better ways to distract or soothe yourself.

• Learn the technique of mindfulness, which helps you witness your negative feelings without engaging with them. Observe them as you would clouds floating by. This will teach you that your thoughts and feelings are not you, just a part of you.

KEY #5

Know What's Enough

• Create a list of what you have "enough of" in life, including friends, money, joy, passion, love, space, self-love, food, freedom, savings, structure, brains, talent, pastimes, possessions, etc. On what basis did you decide that you have a sufficient amount? Notice how sufficiency is a felt sense.

• Make a list of what you don't have enough of in your life. On what basis did you decide that there's a deficit? Quantify your deficit, that is, how much more would you need to achieve sufficiency? A lot, a little? How do you know this?

• What do you tell yourself that you're deprived of that in reality you have enough of? What causes you to misspeak this way?

• Make a list of things you have too much of in reality, including possessions, friends, workload, commitments, space, freedom, or structure. On what basis did you decide that you have too much?

Quantify your "excess," that is, how much less would you need to achieve a sense of sufficiency?

• What were you deprived of in childhood or earlier in life? Were they tangible or intangible? Can you get enough of them now? What would be enough?

• Where do you feel deprivation in your body? Next time you feel deprived, tend to the physical sensations until the emotion goes away.

• Spend a meal or food interaction focusing on when you've had enough in terms of quantity. How did you know that? Be specific.

• Spend a meal or food interaction focusing on quality and identify the peak moment you reach satisfaction. How did you know when it arrived?

• Make a list of your irrational beliefs about deprivation, sufficiency, and deservedness, and reframe them to rational.

• Every day pay attention to what is enough in whatever you're doing, whether it's eating, relaxing, working, playing with the kids, or watching TV. Notice how you know you're approaching or have reached a saturation point. Keep your mind and body tuned into The Sufficiency Channel 24/7.

• Notice when you feel deserving or undeserving. When you feel the latter, remind yourself that you're deserving 100% of the time.

• Catch yourself when you start to make decisions from entitlement, then remind yourself that there are far better ways to decide what you want.

• Observe how other people make decisions and see if you can catch them making decisions based on entitlement. Listen for the words, "because I deserve it."

KEY #6

Manage Intimacy

• Whenever you're with people, notice if you wish to be closer to them emotionally or would like more distance. Do they give you enough physical and emotional space? Do they dominate the conversation? Do they pull away from you as you move closer to them? Do you pull away from them as they move closer to you?

• Monitor when you feel most sexual: with certain people, in specific situations, at home, in public, hormonally, in particular clothes, at what time of day or night, and under what conditions. When you're out and about, notice whom you are attracted to and identify what causes the attraction.

• Which celebrities turn you on physically? Emotionally? What is it about them?

• What makes someone turn you off emotionally or physically? Is this something they can change or is it a permanent feature of their appearance or personality?

• Select someone you'd like to know better as a friend and inch toward that happening—initiate a conversation, spend a bit more time than usual talking with them, invite them for coffee or a walk. Notice their reaction.

• Select someone you'd like to have more distance from and incrementally work toward that happening—have shorter or less frequent phone calls, leave an interaction early, share less about yourself, and be less involved in their drama.

• Notice if intimacy and sexuality go hand in hand or whether you're attracted to people with whom you don't feel much intimacy.

• Make a list of the qualities which make you attracted to someone and then decide if these are worthy attributes or not. You might find that you like "bad boys" or "ice queens."

• Create a family chart going back to your grandparents or great-grandparents and write what you know about their ability to be intimate. This will help you understand why you are the way you are.

• Make a list of what prevents you from being more intimate with people: fears, addictions, beliefs, values, tight schedule, friends, or family.

• What qualities are you looking for in friends?

• Which of the qualities you are looking for in friends and lovers do you have? Which ones can you acquire? How hard will that be and how will you do it?

• Make a list of your irrational beliefs about intimacy and sexuality and reframe them to rational.

• Search magazines and the Internet for sexually attractive people and people in love who may be larger than the norm.

• As a friend of mine who had a double mastectomy proudly proclaims, "My sexuality is between my ears." Is yours?

• Stop looking in magazines at "beautiful" people and stop watching any and all make-over TV shows. They will only make you feel less desirable than you are. Find something more worthwhile and constructive to do with your time—something that will add value to your life and to the world.

• When you're alone, try feeling sexual. Act out a scenario in your head of seducing someone or being seduced. First do it in the dark, next do it with a light on. Keep track of your reactions to these experiences. Repeat as needed until you're more comfortable with your body and feeling sexual.

• Read erotic literature and allow yourself to be turned on. Masturbate.

• Understand how you regulate intimacy or sexuality. Do you speak your mind, expect others to read it, or let your body give off signals you hope will be interpreted correctly? Experiment with saying what turns you on and off. If an experiment at expressing yourself directly fails, keep on speaking up until you're comfortable.

• Make a list of the messages about sexuality and intimacy you've internalized from family, media, religion, and culture. Go through the list with a fine tooth-comb to see which ones you want to hold on to and which to toss away now that you can think for yourself.

• Try wearing less or more sexy clothing depending on how you usually dress. It's okay to be a little uncomfortable; in fact, that's the point of this experiment, to stretch yourself. Ditto with make-up: if you usually wear gobs, go without or tone it down and if you never wear any, dab some on. Then leave the house.

• Get a massage. Ask a friend for a recommendation. If you're anxious, have a bit of wine before you go (not too much or you'll spend all your time in the bathroom rather than on the massage table). Share the fact that you're uncomfortable with the person giving you the massage. It won't be anything new to them.

• Observe the images people project, both strangers and folks you know. Practice noticing who is authentic (you can usually sense it) and isn't putting on a persona to please or impress you.

• Make a list of how relationships might change when you're thinner or fatter.

KEY #7

Develop a Healthy Identity

• Make a list of your favorite and least-liked TV, movie, or fiction characters and describe their identities, for example, always looking for a fight, tough on the outside and mush on the inside, screws everything up, etc.

• Make a list of your favorite and least-liked historical or current political figures, describing how they come across and what draws you to them or puts you off, for example, flip-flopper, know-it-all, blowhard, people-pleaser, etc.

• Brainstorm all your personas—personal and professional--and don't stop until you really can't think of any more.

• Write about how you'd act at different weights than you are now at work, with family, at a party, and interacting with strangers. How much different would you be if weight wasn't a concern? How much the same?

• Do you hide the best part of you who are? What is that part? Make a point of showing it to someone this week.

• From your body language, words, tone of voice, and style, what image do you project? What percentage of you is really like that? What are your other sub-identities?

• If you've been a victim, are you still projecting that image? Ask other people you trust. Yes, that's a scary thing to do, but how else will you ever know the truth?

• Monitor how you act around people. Are you the same no matter what group you're in or do you have different personas for different people?

• Make a list of what will absolutely, positively not change about you even if you give up some of the ways you project yourself. You might want to give up playing a victim, struggling, showing people that you've suffered, being envious, trying to be perfect. Say you chuck 'em all, what will still be left that's truly you?

• Make a list of pros and cons about feeling visible or invisible.

• Make a list of your irrational beliefs about your identity and reframe them to rational.

• Make a list of what's true about your persona no matter what your weight.

• Go to a place where you don't know people and try projecting a different image. If you're usually a laugh a minute, be serious; if you tend to talk about yourself, ask questions. Notice how strangers react to you. Now try this same exercise with acquaintances and work your way up to people you know well. I promise you won't be arrested for impersonation.

About the Author

Karen R. Koenig, LCSW, M.Ed, is a psychotherapist, international eating coach, national educator, and popular author of five books on eating and weight. She is an expert on the psychology of eating—the how and why, not the what of it—and is best known for her non-diet, "normal" eating approach to making peace with food. She has worked in the field of eating disorders for 30 years.

Her books include: *The Rules of "Normal" Eating* (2005) and *The Food & Feelings Workbook* (2007) published by Gürze Books, as well as *What Every Therapist Needs to Know about Treating Eating and Weight Issues* (Norton Professional Books, 2008), and *Nice Girls Finish Fat* (Simon and Schuster, 2009). Among three of her books, there are 10 foreign language translations.

Ms. Koenig practices in Sarasota, Florida, moderates an online Food and Feelings message board, and blogs at *www. EatingDisordersBlogs.com/healthy.*

Her website is *www.karenkoenig.com.*